Push NOW!

Push NOW!

Stories from the Delivery Room

Dana Hoffer

Push NOW!

Language editing: Joy Pincus
Cover design: Noa Gold
Cover photo: Orit Segal
Translated from the Hebrew by Idan Haim

Moments publishing
Ma'ale Zvia, Israel
Hoffer.dana@gmail.com

ISBN-13: 9781522999140
ISBN-10: 1522999140

First edition 2016

Acknowledgements

I would like to thank the people who assisted in delivering this book into the world:

To Ethra McKay, the representative of a special trio, who have made my life far richer and closer to being as human life was meant to be.

To Dani Davidi, a gate opener, a mind opener, and a heart opener. A man through which many of the perceptions that wrote this book has arrived.

To the Future Forward fund, for its generous support, which enabled the translation of this book into English. Thanks for your faith and trust in the book and in me.

To my friend, Sharon Call-Or, who has read the book again and again, and when she was done smiling and crying, sent her invaluable remarks, thereby helping to make the book much better.

To my friends, Ruti Gal, Yael Avner and Amir Call-Or, whose perceptions and remarks were important and enlightening.

To Joy Pincus, for the wonderful linguistic editing, which made an Israeli woman from the Galilee sound like a New Yorker.

To Liliane Oks, for promoting the processing of publishing the book in its English version, and for the support and accompaniment along this long and winding adventure.

To the dear staff of my delivery room. I learn so much from each and every one of you and feel lucky to have you as my partners in this never-ending, life-changing journey.

To all the women in labor, thank you for allowing me to share with you one of the most significant times of your life. It is a great privilege for me to be there with you at these moments.

To Eitan, my partner, and to my children, for the support, love and daily lessons I receive while living alongside you.

"So, you're a midwife? What a lovely profession!"

That's more or less the basic response of most people when they hear that I'm a midwife. They never understand why I don't rush to agree with them, and why, in fact, a little scowl creeps over my face. Yes, my profession is perhaps the most fascinating subject in the world, at least to me; yes, almost every day I am present to usher in the arrival of a new life into this world. And yes, I also witness many tears of joy and lots of love and excitement all around me, but I also see many other things. It's not because I am a "glass half empty" kind of person, but rather that I'm just not afraid to look.

When I'm not afraid to look, I see that a birth is not always the highlight in the life of a happily-married couple. Sometimes a marriage is not really happy. Sometimes a pregnancy is not really desirable; and sometimes it is just plain unwanted.

When I'm not afraid to look, I see those women who are so anxious at the prospect of giving birth. Some are just afraid of the pain, which is inseparable from the birth process, but others, a large proportion actually if you check the statistics, were sexually abused as children, and giving birth, for them, is like opening Pandora's box. I also see how abused women look at their husbands to seek approval before answering the doctor's questions. Women's medical charts tell me their medical history, and I learn about the miscarriages, the abortions and the disabled children that are sometimes waiting at home. Sometimes, and I'm thankful that it's only rarely, I also companion women at the birth of stillborn babies.

A delivery room is not only a place of happiness and joy, flowers and butterflies. For some women, it's a scary place, one they do not want to be in; for others, it's where they yearn to reach, but never will.

Birth itself is far from being a romantic process, with a pink baby wrapped in lacy white linen waiting at the end. During birth there is pain, fear, power, blood, vomit, feces, tears, despair, hope, joy, wild excitement and unruly behavior. Or, sometimes, there is complete silence, confusion and uncertainty. All of this is mixed together over many hours and only then do you get to see your pink baby swaddled in lace; sometimes not even then.

So, no -- I wouldn't call it a "lovely" profession. An exciting profession? Yes. Challenging? Definitely. This is a profession that enables me every day to learn a great deal about people, and even more about myself - my weaknesses, abilities, fears, prejudices and strengths.

A delivery room is a place of wonders for me, a place of experience; but above all, a delivery room is home to me. This book is basically a travelogue: a journey that begins in the School of Midwifery and continues through my first years as a midwife. Today, when I read what I wrote back then, I find it hard to resist the urge to rewrite all the nonsense I once thought. I also have a longing within to feel things the way I once did. But that's part of what I love about my profession – that I encounter people at one of the most powerful moments in their lives - and this touches me, changes me... reshapes me every time.

So how did I, who once dreamed of becoming a veterinarian, who did not say the word "period" out loud until the age of twenty-six, who would always blush when I saw a couple kissing in the cinema, and who often felt shy, even in front of people I knew; how did I find myself in what is truly the oldest profession in the world?

And so the journey begins...

So I've finally started to study midwifery; after several years of dreams, three years of nursing school, one year in college and one year working as a nurse, I'm embarking on this journey equipped with everything I need: Hopes, dreams, ideas, worries, desires, knowledge, ignorance, fear, confidence and joy - the whole nine yards.

I'm embarking on a journey that winds itself through every nook and cranny of the Israeli healthcare system – towards which my feelings shift between mild dislike and deep revulsion, depending on what time of day I might be asked. The healthcare system, with all its faults and virtues, approaches many issues in ways that are diametrically opposed to how I believe they should be handled. It's a system that is hard to live with. Nevertheless, I'm embarking on this journey and I wish myself *bon voyage.*

❖ ❖ ❖

The first three days of the course are over. The lectures were interesting and the knowledge has begun to flow and wash over me, in slow, little trickles at first, but one can hear and feel the raging flood that is coming. I find myself in eager anticipation; my brain **loves** to know things; it loves to ask questions, investigate and discover.

And the lecturers amaze me, too. Whenever they are asked about the purpose of a certain organ they answer, "And who said this organ has a purpose? To say it has a purpose implies someone designed us!" But the mysteries of our body and its wonders amaze me anew every time and, the way I see it, don't leave a lot of room for doubt regarding the existence of a grand design.

One lecturer annoyed me a bit. He claimed that it is every woman's right to give birth by Caesarean section, even if there is no medical reason for it, and if we do not allow her to have this procedure, then we are really "forcing" her to give birth against her will (Excuse me? Are we the ones who got her pregnant?) forcing her to face the possible complications of birth, the dangers of birth, the pain of birth, the possible complications, possible problems and complications, not to mention the difficulties and... oh, did we mention complications? Someone might think that a Caesarean section is simple and easy and without complications...

So I thought to myself, maybe I'll go to a good surgeon and tell him I'm sick of this whole idea of going to the toilet. Maybe he can just hook me up with a stoma[1] instead? And if he refuses, then I'll just tell him that he is denying me the right to decide about my own body. Ugh!

It seems that almost none of the other students are oriented towards natural birth. Most of them shake their heads and sigh when someone mentions a home birth. One actually said in astonishment, "How can a birth even take place if the woman isn't connected to a monitor[2]?" It's a wonder that humanity survived until the advent of the monitor.

---

1 Stoma – an artificial opening in the abdominal wall designed to drain the intestinal contents in patients where part of the colon has been surgically removed.

2 Fetal Monitor- the evaluation of the condition of the fetus during pregnancy and childbirth takes place via a number of tools: a sense of movement by the mother, ultrasound and a fetal monitor. The monitor records the FHR, (fetal heart rate) and contractions, if there are any. The midwife or doctor interprets the monitor's chart and according to it estimates the condition of the baby. When everything in the chart seems OK, the meaning is that the baby is OK.

I wonder if the short duration of the course (nine weeks of theory, and then a hop, skip and a jump, straight to internship) even allows for a change in perception. Is there any chance of opening the eyes of some of the women there, who in just one year will start helping other women deliver? Perhaps yes, but I also remind myself that changes need time to percolate, and that too-sudden changes often turn out to fleeting ones that don't last the distance. I too once gave fiery speeches about those irresponsible women who want a natural birth, and while I've changed, this transformation didn't happen overnight.

When something in the chart is out of order, only in 30% of cases it means that something is actually wrong with the baby, most babies still feel fine. The use of a monitor raised the caesarean section rate due to 'fetal distress' but did not improve mortality or morbidity in infants. Nevertheless, there is still no tool with a higher level of accuracy that can continuously give information about the baby's condition during labor.

The second week of studies

Today we had a great lecture on the history of midwifery, with lots of beautiful pictures of women who gave birth naked, strong and beautiful... ancient goddesses, round and voluptuous. One big understanding dawned on me: once people began to intervene in pregnancies - and yes, we began to intervene long, long ago, maybe two thousand years or more - things just got worse. The more doctors intervened, the more there were problems, infections and mortality. But when there were only midwives, or when they served only poor women who could not afford a doctor, the situation was always better.

This peaked in the late 19th century, with the mortality rate of women in hospital maternity wards reaching 35%, and up to 80% for women who contracted an infection during their stay. That lasted until someone named Dr. Semmelweis thought that perhaps he should wash his hands when going from examining rotting cadavers to delivering babies in the maternity ward. His hospital mortality rates decreased to just a few percent, yet his ideas were soundly rejected by his peers.

Another significant realization I had regarding natural childbirth is that we have deviated from the proper path for so many years that getting back on the right track is almost impossible, simply because no one remembers what the original and natural way to give birth is, anymore. A bit more uplifting was the thought that, actually, despite all the interventions that take place in the Western world, there are still millions of Native Americans and African women who give birth naturally. Someone was still managing to keep the embers burning, despite the bleak situation of Europe, where thousands of years of ancient knowledge were being thrown away.

It turns out that the conflict between midwives and doctors did not begin in the last hundred years, but has been around for centuries. No wonder it's so hard to create good, effective and healing relationships between them. It's not just a matter of building a pleasant working environment; it's to do with coming to a meeting of minds, or at least mutual respect for each other's opinions about even the smallest details of treatment. Is it possible to turn over a new leaf and start anew? I suppose so… I hope so.

After arriving home at the end of this long day of studies, I went for a walk in my neighborhood, an urban jungle of high-rise buildings and concrete. As I reached the end of the street, the Shomron Mountains were revealed in the distance, and as my eyes reached up towards these open horizons, I felt my mind begin to fly as well. It enabled me to reach more deeply inside myself, and I began to think about midwifery and why I feel such a deep sense of calling for this profession. From which part of me does it emanate – this drive, this desire, this urge and need to be there, with those women giving birth? The answer to this question is still forming, and it is too early to tell, but I hope it will reveal itself in time.

Meanwhile, in the maternity ward where I'm working

A new mother is admitted to the ward after giving birth. Her medical chart describes the event:

'Artificial rupture of the amniotic membranes, labor induced with Pitocin, epidural anesthesia, episiotomy incision, sewing of incision.' Finally, the concluding diagnosis: *'spontaneous delivery'*[3]

And I think to myself, "spontaneous delivery!" What on earth was so spontaneous about it?

3 Spontaneous delivery is the accepted term for an ordinary vaginal delivery.

Back in the classroom

An amazing course in Embryology[4]: First a sperm and an egg... then a single cell that divides into two, four, eight, and then a million... cells that form the brain, kidneys, skin, muscles, uterus. Each cell knows exactly what to do, reporting to its pre-designated position without any argument; the work of God on Earth. And someone behind me mutters:

"Remind me why exactly we need to learn this?"

Another lecturer teaches about the menstrual cycle. According to his explanation, hormones burst into colorful dances, which are far more complicated than any perceivable tango. The endometrium, which is the mucous membrane of the uterus, mimics the legendary phoenix: it is born, develops, falls out, and gets born again. All pieces of the puzzle fit perfectly; there are no extraneous parts or redundancies. And someone asks:

"Are you telling me this cycle happens every month?"

I know that I sound a bit frustrated... even very frustrated. Indeed, I'm having a hard time understanding why some of my classmates have chosen this profession. Some of the students have asked me how it is that I know so much. As in knowing that the **monthly** cycle happens **every month**...? I'm practically speechless. It's not I who knows so much, it is they who know so little, and have even less interest in learning.

Beyond that, I don't feel around me the love for those pregnant women giving birth. One professor stated in class, during a

4 Embryology – the science of embryo development in the womb.

discussion regarding conflicts between midwives and doctors, that: "We all know that the real enemy is actually the woman in labor." He received a tremendous ovation and was quoted extensively for days afterward… I was not amused, even if it was only a joke.

I have very quickly gained the reputation of someone who is a bit of a freak. After speaking out that maybe it is not necessary to make seven ultrasound scans in a normal pregnancy (oddly enough gaining the support of the lecturing doctor), one of the students told me that for all she cared I could go right now and give birth at home, eat organic food all day and sing to the stars. Well, obviously this is not a real insult. To me, it sounds more like a dream come true.

I am acutely aware, as the weeks pass and the course progresses in giant leaps and bounds, that it's all heading towards our practical experience. It is hard for me to think about anything else, and even that big examination that's coming up doesn't really bother me. I'm mostly afraid of one thing: that I will drop a baby. I have told myself over and over again how silly this is, and that I've actually never heard of a midwife who dropped a baby. But in the back of my head, I see myself as a seven year old, opening the refrigerator door, pouring milk with trembling hands into a glass on the counter and dropping the carton on the floor. I remember my father's scolding voice telling me, "You've got two left hands."

This is nonsense, of course. One has only to look at my hands to see that I do in fact have two opposing thumbs. So, in light of such evidence, I clearly have only one left hand. And while as a child I was indeed clumsy, and yes a bit of that has been retained in me today, it never turns up for things that are important to me. For example, I've never dropped the violin of my beloved partner, Eitan. I have also never dropped a baby. I paint pretty well, and I try to crochet every once in a while. I cut vegetables for salad without slicing my fingers, most of the time, and I give injections in the right places. People even tell me they really don't hurt.

My fears are substantiated, however, by the combination of slick rubber gloves, a baby covered with slippery vernix[5] and born over a bed where the lower part has been broken down, positioning him straight over the gaping chasm below... no one could argue with me that it would be a lot safer if the mother gave birth squatting on a mattress on the floor, or in water.

I told Judy, a midwife who gave us some eye-opening lectures during the course, about my concerns, hoping of course that she would calm me down ("What a bunch of nonsense, come on!") But she actually confirmed my suspicions: "Yes, it really is very scary..." This, of course, frightened me even more. And while Judy went on to give me some practical advice on how to hold the baby and how to avoid dropping it, I'm still afraid... especially since the first hospital in which I will be practicing will probably insist that first-time mothers in labor deliver their babies over a disassembled bed[6], i.e., the baby will come out over a trash can placed strategically at the foot of the bed.

Oh well, maybe it is better that he falls into the bin and not straight onto the floor?

When I'm not studying, I work as a nurse in the maternity ward, where there is no room for these kinds of thoughts. The hospital's routine obliterates everything. Everyone is now busy worrying about Miriam, the head nurse of the labor ward. Last year she had cancer, then she broke her leg, and now she's recently broken her arm. "How did that happen?" I asked curiously.

---

5 Vernix – a rubbery white substance that covers the skin of the fetus during pregnancy and protects it.

6 In some hospitals, the lower part of a hospital bed is disassembled right before birth to turn it into a gynecologist's bed. The woman's legs rest in special stirrups and the baby comes out straight into the hands of the midwife, with nothing but the floor underneath him.

"Oh, she went over to weigh a baby after birth, slipped on a puddle of amniotic fluid and fell with the baby in her arms."

"And the baby?" I cried.

"Huh, he's fine. But Miriam broke her arm, the poor thing…"

I need a moment to calm down. Or maybe not; fear has proven itself a good ally so far.

One step away from the real thing

Today we played with dolls. We tested their cervical dilation and cervical effacement, as well as the position of their babies' heads. We supported them emotionally and analyzed their monitor charts. One poor doll had to give birth thirty-one times today (and you think you had a difficult birth?). It was a fun and exciting day.

Of course, I delivered the doll five times, which is four times more than I should have, and guess what? I didn't drop the baby, not even once! On the contrary, I held him in a safe and firm grip and set him down at his mother's breast. I even had a situation with one baby (which actually was the same poor baby over and over), where the umbilical cord was wrapped around his neck. I loosened the cord with a skilled hand and saved him from irreversible brain damage.

In short, it was a day full of small and amusing victories. Of course, I don't actually think that I know how to deliver a real baby, not yet, but I still feel a bit better.

Tomorrow we have a test, and next week it's the delivery room!

I think I chose the right profession. Everything I'm experiencing seems to me to be the greatest things in the world! The only problem I foresee in my coming practice is that I am not allowed to stay at work for more than ten hours a day…

But I am also afraid. I'm afraid of my disagreement with the establishment and its procedures and opacity; I'm afraid I'll have to make unnecessary interventions and examinations that have no purpose other than to cover my rear end; I'm afraid of my lack of experience and my ignorance; I'm afraid of working with emotionless, obtuse doctors or midwives; afraid of the powerful internal conflict that I know will come. There's no chance it won't. After all, as one gets more deeply involved in this field, these conflicts become more and more critical. It is I who will have to cut the unnecessary episiotomy, and my eyes that will have to analyze the unnecessary monitor, and my voice that will have to call the sometimes unnecessary doctor. Sometimes I ask myself what I am even getting myself into. This system will force me to do things that I don't always agree with, or with the rationale behind them.

I know that, on the other hand, it is good that I'll be there to counter all these reasons. As well, I am aware that these actions are not always unnecessary. They are sometimes life saving and beneficial and very much necessary. In short, it is an inner conflict. And despite the clashes and battles that I am anticipating, I expect I will experience them with a true and open heart.

And I'm already there in the delivery room

The practical experience element of a midwifery course includes working in two different hospitals, for three months each. Thankfully, none of these hospitals is the one I work in as a nurse. This way, I will have a chance to be exposed to different work methods. I am supposed to attend at least fifty births and help with several Caesarean sections, as well as some assisted deliveries.

This week I spent three intense days in the delivery room of the hospital where I started my first session of practical experience, and now I'm trying to organize in my head all that I saw and did there. There is so much to tell, and so much to think about, to understand, to learn from. This will be an ongoing story…

Orientation

It starts with a tour of the ward, or in other words, an "Orientation Round." There's a reception room, labor rooms and a Jacuzzi which to me looked more like a regular bathtub; along with four delivery rooms, one of which even has a balcony with lovely views of mountains and valleys. There's also a nursing station with lots of cabinets that contain equipment like needles and syringes, medicines, disinfectants, towels, containers, all kinds of forms, test tubes, gloves, belts, oxygen masks and myriad other things, some familiar and some new.

With every cabinet that opens or electrical appliance that someone demonstrates I get a little more stressed, and think to myself that just to learn what every button on every device does would take a month. And when do I even start to learn how to deliver a baby?

But then I calm down and tell myself firmly: "Dana, please, don't worry, you'll learn everything faster than you think. You can deal with any difficulty or with any new thing thrown at you." And oddly enough, this helps, and on the second day it seems that there aren't so many forms, or syringes, or instruments with buttons.

The staff

The staff welcomes me warmly and graciously. They invite me for coffee and cookies, ask about where and how, and how much time, and why, and who do I know that they know too, and so on – in fact, after a couple of minutes they're already passing on their regards to distant acquaintances. And they offer encouragement, promising me that I will have a fun and interesting time, and soon enough I feel quite at home, or at least like I'm back in my old ward.

My first delivery

On the first day of my practical experience, there is a full staff - four midwives, one nurse, two nursing students and me. This venerable ensemble meets only a single patient.

I immediately find myself in the delivery room with a lovely midwife, who has been on the job more years than I have lived. The mother is an Arab woman, so I feel even more at home when I speak Arabic to her. Lately I've started thinking in Arabic, since it is the main language spoken at the hospital where I work as a nurse. The birth is the mother's first delivery, and it is a long, long, long one. How can I describe it in one shot? Well, maybe like this:

Sedatives, a suspect monitor, induction of labor, feeling lonely, another attempt to induce labor, a stressful doctor, shouting, stress, ten people in the room, "I'll give you the vacuum!" fear, pressure, episiotomy, bleeding, the baby is out, getting the baby straight to the nursery, a tired mother, a doctor stitches, mother without a baby drinking tea in the hall.

I feel quite depressed after this day. The slippery slope of intervention that everyone is always talking about is so scary when you meet it face to face. When you see clearly how one small intervention leads to a slightly larger intervention and how from there you're just sliding, with no way to stop. And how from a normal birth with a healthy baby and a healthy mother, every possible pathology can develop; and how one puts the pressure on and gets stressed out, scares and becomes scared, discourages and gets discouraged.

I know that no one had bad intentions. On the contrary, everyone wanted to help the delivery and the baby, and it was important to everyone that mother and baby were safe and sound at the end of the delivery. And yet, everything could have turned out differently. This is something that keeps echoing in my head - how it all could have turned out differently. And how the mother of the woman that is giving birth had done the same in her home, or perhaps, being a Bedouin, in her tent, and how she gave birth to eight healthy children there, and why is it that our culture has created such a terrible monster?

Next up: my second birth.

Warning: it is quite similar to the first one.

My second birth

A new day arrives, and again there are a lot of staff and only one mother in the delivery room – in fact, she is the wife of a good friend of mine from nursing school, who was admitted to have her labor induced, because her doctor scared her that terrible things might happen if she didn't. I advise her to run away back home as fast as she can, but it will take her another twenty-four hours to reach this conclusion on her own. In the meantime, I join the crowd in the delivery room and this time the drama unfolds as follows:

First attempt at an epidural, second attempt at an epidural, partially successful epidural, "Let me give you an enema. You should! It's really recommended! You have to!" And intravenous fluids, and a monitor, and a blood pressure gauge, and a urinary catheter, and "Let's get your water to break – it will make everything really fast. I recommend it. You don't want to? Never mind, I already did it. It's really recommended!"

And oops, there is meconium in the amniotic fluid, so we'll connect a monitor to the baby's head, and "No, you can't really change positions, because if you try to move to the right you'll see the epidural catheter is too short, and if you try to move to the left the IV fluids may come out. It's best that you lie on your back and just rest for a while."

And here the baby comes out, "Push, harder! Harder! Don't push, push, don't push, push! Now, now, now! Congratulations!"

And again I think to myself - how it all could have turned out differently.

Next up - the third day, in which there were three births. Note: a corrective experience.

The third day

On the third day, it is clear from the beginning that things are going to be different. As soon as I get there, a midwife sticks her head out from a delivery room and calls me to join her. And so, straight from home, from the outside world, I am pulled straight into another world - the world of birth, where I stay until the afternoon. There's no need to go deeply into stories of all three labors; just a few little things: three mothers, three different worlds. I already know that everyone is different, unique and special, but it is astounding to see how much of this is expressed at birth!

One woman in labor comes in with a smile, and says, "I always give birth with an 8-centimeter dilation," smiles and gives birth with no analgesic or medication. While she is breastfeeding in the delivery room, I receive a warm invitation from her lovely mother and mother-in-law to visit them in their village.

The second woman in labor is highly withdrawn between contractions, totally in her own world. But at the right moment, she springs into action and gives birth to her baby.

And the third woman in labor is wild, upset, hurt, raging...but finally she gives birth, becoming a mother for the first time.

And with two of the three births, those had been my hands supporting and helping the baby to come into the world. To my delight, my instructor's hands were there with me. What a relief! Oddly enough, no baby fell, no midwife dropped anything, and all's well that ends well.

The delivery of my 16th baby

It would actually be more accurate to say that its mother delivered her, and that this baby girl made her way out. I just happened to be there.

It begins with a mother who wants to try a natural birth, and a delivery room too busy for anyone to tell her otherwise, including me (as it turns out, it seems that I am sometimes amazingly and intentionally slow in following instructions). You know how long it takes me to give a woman an enema and get her into the delivery room? Sometimes two hours. It turns out that given the time and opportunity, freed of any stress or demands, the body somehow knows how to do the job on its own. A little patience in the delivery room could save a lot of unnecessary interventions – and just to be fair, this lack of patience does not always emanate from doctors and midwives. Sometimes it's the woman giving birth who is too impatient to wait for it to just happen, and sometimes it's the husband, who is dying to go home already.

This woman walks around for most of the birth, and in the last two hours, after she returns to the delivery room, she is absorbed in her own world, with only the pain of the contractions penetrating its veil. But even during her contractions, she does not open her eyes, but just moves restlessly in bed. Between contractions she just floats in that world. Then she begins to push, and since Na'ama, my instructor, gives me quite a lot of leeway (or as she puts it, "Just imagine I died, and in the meantime I'll do an impression of an armchair"), I do not intervene or instruct her on how to push and for how long.

After a while, I feel something is stuck so I call Na'ama. Second births usually advance much faster than first births, but even though she is pushing and pushing, nothing is happening. Na'ama suggests that the woman turn over onto her hands and knees. Two contractions in this position, and hop, she lies on her back again and, with a river of clear amniotic fluid spilling directly on me, of course, the baby emerges into this world. Such a sweetie! The moment I put her on her mother's abdomen, she opens her huge eyes in astonishment, as if to say, "Hello world, I have arrived." Within a few minutes she is sucking vigorously, and this sight, for me at that moment, is the most beautiful thing in the world.

Please understand; this is an abbreviated story of just one birth. I have another six like it from last week alone. Some births are beautiful and some make me cry inside, because they represent so many missed opportunities and stupidity and ignorance. Many times, I feel that the ignorance is mine. I weep for knowledge lost in time; a position that would help a particular baby come out; a forgotten song to calm an anxious mother; an herb that can speed up contraction...all the lost wisdom of days gone by. I know that a lot of it has been collected these days, and we are aware of and study some of it, but just how much of what was lost have we really managed to find?

And then there is the pain, which clearly holds a secret and has power... but how? Of what nature? I still do not have the exact answer, and perhaps I never will, but I feel it. I feel the power that is present when I meet a room full of pain; it is a pool filled to the brim with pain, and without shying away and closing the door, or running to hide in a distant corner, instead I enter and close the door behind me, jump into this pool and let the quiet and dark water envelop and swallow me, without fear. At first, it takes my breath away and something inside me shrinks. It is difficult to be in the presence of pain; pure and raw, without painkillers, unmasked, where only it exists. But then, if one does not shy away, breathing becomes regular again, and one can offer solace from a different place, somewhere more pure. Not from a place of fear, of wishing the pain to go away, but from a place of love and companionship.

And it's hard to overcome this urge to try and ease the pain, to make it go away. It's hard to just stay with it. Sometimes I feel that I have to fight an enormous impulse inside of me – similar to the impulse that makes us offer someone a tissue when they are crying instead of just letting them cry as much as they need.

But out from this pain, which is just pain after all, there grows such power and such wonderful savagery, that all of one's hidden capabilities suddenly rise up and become real. The experience takes shape, something one can sink one's teeth into, and taste and smell, as opposed to the pain-free experience, which is completely bland. Not painful, but also not very exciting. It does not touch that exposed nerve inside.

And this is true for anything, not just birth. I think it's a trick of the world that makes us miss a lot of life's nectar, the real taste of life. Because we always run away from tough experiences, run away from pain and fear, and blood and death. We are afraid of life. But real life is not found in sterile rooms, or under bright fluorescent lights. Real life is found in our homes.

Real life happens at home

Real life happens at home. This phrase crossed my mind many times over the past month, during which I spent time with a good friend who was dying. And that was indeed like a home "birth" – very special. The whole farewell process constantly reminded me of the difference between giving birth in the hospital and giving birth at home, and just how much real life happens at home.

And by "home" I don't mean just the house or apartment where we live; I'm referring more to the natural environment in which things occur. Whether at home, in a garden, on a mountain top or just walking down the street, only in their natural environment can things happen as they're meant to, the way we want them to, which leads to decisions that are based in logical and natural considerations.

For a while now, I've been thinking about the name of my profession. In Hebrew, nurses are called sisters. Why do they use this word, and not 'healer' or 'physician assistant ' or something else? Some people claim this comes from the nuns,[7] who were the first to function as nurses, but I think it has to do with the fact that long ago, a pregnant woman or a sick man were treated at home by their family: brothers, sisters, children, parents and cousins. Every person encountered births, illnesses, and deaths long before they entered the adult world and these things were accepted as just another part of life. It was one of the most important messages my friend who passed away tried to convey to everyone around him – do not fear.

"Death is not frightening, but rather a gift and an opportunity. If you could only understand that," he repeated, "then your life would

7 In convents, nuns are also referred to as 'sisters'.

be totally different, filled with love instead of fear." Ever since, this message has remained with me and I have no fear.

This friend almost died several times in the weeks before his passing. On each of these occasions, he spoke of having "one foot in the next world" and that he saw and felt what awaited him in the afterlife. After these encounters, he was no longer afraid of death, but happily waiting for it. He also made sure that there was nothing left unsaid, to anyone. He talked freely about everything, and this was a gift to many people. He died in peace, and that peace continues to surround his home and his family even to this day.

It could have been thus for any one of us, but our culture has become more efficient, and has learned to expertly handle large numbers of people, to save many lives and to prevent suffering and disability. All great, but the price of this professionalism and expertise is, ironically, that very expertise and professionalism. For if you want to treat a sick person today, you need a nurse (preferably with a bachelor's degree) or a specialist, and hospitals with special beds and expensive drugs and devices.

An average person might not encounter serious sickness or death and certainly not birth, until later in life, simply because society has distanced these things from the public eye. Almost no seriously ill people are treated at home, almost no one dies at home and very few women give birth at home. These aspects of life have been exiled to hospitals, where they have been sterilized and neutered. It is a bit like the difference between a canned pineapple and a fresh one. Someone who has never eaten the real thing doesn't know what he's missing.

An important note: I too was born in a hospital, I have friends whose lives were saved or drastically improved by modern medicine, and I can't, or won't, imagine life today without it. I only note to myself the price we pay for this, and carefully examine the limits of possible change.

The delivery of the 17th baby - hers, not mine

A woman is giving birth for the seventeenth time. Her seventeenth! This means sixteen children at home - eight boys and eight girls. Sixteen!

My goodness! Imagine the practical aspects of running a household with sixteen children, soon to be seventeen; I get tired just thinking about it. And this woman is totally relaxed, organized, manicured, not really taking part in all the excitement surrounding her "unusual situation." She is just being who she is: a mother who has come to deliver her baby, that's all.

Na'ama tells me that women who have given birth many times usually have a slow birth, just like first-timers. The uterus has been stretched and contracted so many times that some of the muscle elasticity is lost, and many times they have births that advance at a very slow pace and can get stuck for hours and hours. But this time there are no worries; the woman was admitted with a dilation of 8 centimeters, and everyone knows that in a couple of seconds the baby will be out.

The woman knows it as well, but there's only one little problem: she refuses to give birth without an epidural.

"Epidural!?" the doctor says, horrified. "We'll never make it. You're going to give birth any second now!"

"Epidural!?" my instructor cracks up. "What do you need it for?"

"Epidural!" says the woman calmly. To show her resolve, she crosses her legs defiantly. Well, we run some blood tests and run fluids and call an anesthesiologist.

"Epidural!?" says the anesthesiologist in anger. "For your 17th labor? Are you crazy!?"

"Epidural" she replies.

So we get an epidural. The anesthesiologist is still in the room finishing writing his notes when the woman says, "**Now** I'm ready to give birth." She pushes once and gives birth. She is so delighted. She and her husband are happily holding the baby, who is breast-feeding, and all is well.

This morning I delivered a stillborn baby

I can't really find the words to sum up this day, but I'll try anyway. This was a hard day, a long day, a painful day. This was an insightful day, a special day, a complex day.

Today I met an amazing woman and a very special family that accepted me, even if only for a few hours, as one of them. Actually, I feel a bit like I've become a permanent member of the family. Maybe that's what happens when you shed tears for a person who is dear to someone else.

It was, as you can probably imagine or perhaps remember, if this has happened to you, a confusing and overwhelming situation for the family involved. The delivery room staff calls this kind of birth a "silent birth," because the monitor that is usually present in the room, making soft and rhythmic sounds, is absent in this case. The staff move quietly when they pass the door, the family whispers, the mother cries softly and so does the father. The midwife cries softly too.

I told them in my broken Arabic that they should feel free to cry loudly too, that their child is dead, and although she has not yet been born, she has still been their child, and that it's okay to grieve. When they cried a little louder, the doctor intervened and said we should call a social worker because she thinks the family looks shaken. It made me rather sad, because I often run into this type of approach, which says it is not so sad when a baby is stillborn. After all, the parents did not know the baby and the mother can get pregnant again right away and forget about the whole thing.

But it's not like that, at least not for a large number of women. My mother had to go through this three times; my husband's mother had this happen to her once, and so did my friend. How did it affect my mother? What pain does she carry in her heart? Mom, if you are reading this, what did it do to you?

Anyway, they cried regardless, and continued to do so for a few hours. The woman giving birth was surrounded by a circle of support and love - her husband, her sisters, her mother, her father and several other family members who were there to support her, but did not enter the room. With each contraction, everyone's hands went out to her, one massaging her back, another her legs, a third placing a wet cloth on her forehead, a fourth kissing her, a fifth whispering words of encouragement. And while this is happening, they all cry. Occasionally, one cries a little louder than the others; sometimes the woman who is giving birth and sometimes someone else. No one ever says, "Don't cry now" or "It's not so bad." There was a lot of love among them. No one left the room during the birth, which lasted all through the morning and up to the afternoon. No one looked away or gave the woman the feeling that she had to deal with this by herself.

There was sadness but not loneliness, and they were a hundred percent there for her; quiet, loving, with no nonsense or empty clichés. All this took place in a corner room, rather than in the delivery room. This is because no one wants the mother and family to be around babies that actually cry after they are born.

When she was fully dilated, I asked the woman if she felt the need to push, and she said: "yes... a little". I called in Na'ama so she would be with me, and in three pushes the woman gave birth to a beautiful baby. Perfect, but dead; with the umbilical cord wrapped around her neck. Was this the reason she had died? Maybe, maybe not. Then the family took her, washed her, dressed her in new clothes they had bought for her, and each in turn held her and kissed her. This was done by the mother as well. I did not cry then, but I cry a little now. They took her picture and talked to her and hugged her and loved her. After two and a half hours, the woman made her peace and the family took the baby home to be buried in the family's graveyard.

And so it ends. And in many ways, this is probably also how it begins. And of this whole day, I think what will stay etched in my memory is the image of the woman, surrounded by the love of her family. [8]

8 Fetal death in the uterus occurs in one out of two hundred births. Common causes of a fetal death are linked to medical problems of the mother (e.g., diabetes, infectious diseases, excessive blood clotting), dysfunction of the placenta, a problem – such as a tight knot – in the umbilical cord and some kind of fetal disease, genetic or chromosomal syndrome. Once the situation has been diagnosed, mostly as a result of the woman not feeling fetal movements, the birth has to be induced, because it may take as many as several weeks before a natural birth occurs. If a few weeks have passed and the woman has yet to go into labor, she may develop a condition called "disseminated intravascular coagulation," a blood clotting disorder that may endanger her life. After the birth, tests are often performed on the fetus and placenta to try and determine the cause of death. The tests include cultures, genetic testing of the fetus and an autopsy. However, in a large number of cases, while the cause is never discovered, the situation will not reoccur with the same woman.

Apparently childbirth is a dangerous thing

Today we learned about preventing infections during birth; a most fascinating and frightening subject. Did you know, for example, that in Israel, pregnant women are not required or encouraged to take tests for hepatitis B or HIV? The strangest part of all this is that delivery room staff, me, for example, are required to undergo blood tests for various diseases, a TB test every few years, and a mandatory vaccination.

Now, which scenario is more likely - that I'll spill my bodily fluids onto the patient's eyes while she gives birth, or vice versa? That I will stab myself with a needle and then accidentally stab the patient, or vice versa?

Clearly, it's a million times more likely that biological material will be transferred from the patient to the midwife or doctor, rather than the other way around. And yet, when I meet a woman in the delivery room, I have no idea if she is a carrier of an infectious disease. So what should I do? Wear a hazmat suit before every birth, like they do when there's an Ebola outbreak? Switch careers and become a telephone operator in a call center? Take out life insurance?

The other side of the coin is not that encouraging either. At a certain point, I realized that all we do is create problems and challenges for ourselves and our patients. For example: if we didn't do so many vaginal examinations during birth (some women undergo twenty examinations during the process), we would reduce the post-partum uterine infection rate to a meager few percent. If women gave birth in an upright position, instead of lying on their backs, and midwives didn't have to stand with their faces in front of the woman's vaginal opening, then midwives wouldn't get amniotic fluid and blood squirted in their faces (that happens in 40% of births!) and they wouldn't have to think about how to protect themselves from all sorts of diseases.

If midwives didn't fiddle about so much with the birthing woman's perineum, and women gave birth in an upright position, there would be less contact of stool with the vagina and fewer postpartum reproductive and urinary system infections.

And this is without even taking into account the strange choice by 99% of women in the country to give birth in the most dangerous, bacteria-infected place on earth -- a hospital.

By the way, I received a gift from one of the midwives; protective goggles. When I got home, I showed them to Eitan and he ruled against them. He claimed they are so scary that the baby would just crawl straight back into the womb. I disagreed and made an impassioned speech in their defense. "What? You want me to get HIV?" I ranted.

The next day I took a shower and Eitan surprised me while wearing these goggles. I was so scared that I screamed, and got the point. Yesterday I returned them. What will be, will be.

Yesterday, there were two beautiful births

The first woman arrived, had a shower and a Jacuzzi bath, came into the delivery room and asked for an epidural. I suggested that I examine her dilation first, and see how close she was to giving birth. So I examined her and she had a dilation of 9 centimeters. She was happy and said, "So I definitely don't want an epidural now."

It was very strange. The mother screamed really loudly during contractions, but she, her sister and I chatted freely in between them, as if we were old friends. Then came another painful contraction, accompanied by consolation and massages, with the soon-to-be mother making low voices, and again, a nice and quiet conversation.

Two nursing students who were there told me that they were really nervous about seeing her in so much pain, but it was only they who got nervous. It is hard to describe the feeling there; it was an odd sort of stillness that even the cries of the other mothers did not disturb. It was a bit like a movie I once saw (I cannot remember its name), where there was a house near a railway line, and every few minutes a train passed by and the room would start shaking. People sitting in the room would stop talking for a moment, and then continue after the train had passed, as if nothing had happened, because they were so used to it.

Approximately half an hour later, she gave birth, really easily and with no tear, cut, or anything problematic. After finishing this birth, I told Na'ama how much fun it had been.

Immediately after this delivery, I was called to receive another woman who had been admitted with an advanced dilation, but too early in her pregnancy. This means that she would give birth prematurely. This was her first birth and she herself was hardly more than a child. I approached her as she was calling her parents, crying her eyes out on the phone and too disoriented to tell them where she was and what was happening. That's how this story started.

After some cheering up and a few hugs from Hana, the wonderful midwife who immediately takes every young woman under her wing and fills the role of her mother, we went into the delivery room, and the woman looked me straight in the eye and said, "Do you think I'll be able to have a natural birth?"

Well, you bet she could, and very much so. Between contractions, she had her eyes closed, and during contractions she made low noises or gave a loud cry, according to what she felt was right. And when her charming baby girl was born, crying and waving her hands, it was incredibly heartwarming. It seems to me that during childbirth, the levels of oxytocin[9] also increase in the midwife's bloodstream. And during a natural birth, they increase even more.

---

9 Oxytocin – also known as the "Love Hormone" – is excreted in the body during an orgasm, it produces contractions during childbirth and helps in the release of milk from the breast during lactation. Environmental conditions that encourage its secretion are privacy, dim light, and a sense of security. However, stress and the feeling of being watched suppress its secretion and this is why so many women who come to the delivery room without contractions swear that back at home they had strong contractions every three minutes. They're right; it's just that getting out of their comfortable and familiar nest at home slightly suppressed the secretion of oxytocin. When they feel safe again, the contractions resume and get stronger.

About judgment

"You keep judging the women you care for," said one of my friends, after I told her about some of my delivery room experiences. "Me???" I asked, resentful immediately. But before I go on, let me tell a short story I once heard from a wise man.[10] A beautiful and elegant woman in England was standing in the street, waiting for her bus to arrive. She seemed like she had just left a beauty salon, with her hair nicely done, nails manicured and wearing an elegant dress. Tip-top, as they say. And as the bus arrived and our fancy lady was about to get on it, suddenly one of the people at the bus stop noticed that, to the heel of her elegant shoe, was stuck the largest dog turd he had ever seen. He called out to her: "Madam, you have a turd stuck to your shoe!" But the lady turned her head, as if she had not heard him, hissed quietly, "Go to hell" and got on the bus with the turd still gracing her shoe, to the delight of everyone on board...

When I first heard this story, I decided to do my best not to be that woman, but rather to be more open to what others have to say, in order to better myself, become more refined and personally developed. I don't want to continue walking around with a turd stuck to my shoe. This was one of these moments, and I had a chance to examine the strength of my decision when meeting real life.

I took a few days to think about it, in an attempt to give her reflection some well-rounded thought, allowing it to simmer and

10 `The Night Watchman`, Gemstone Press

mature a bit inside me before coming to any conclusions. Actually, first I took some time to feel deeply insulted, deny her accusation vigorously and stew in anger about the whole thing. But when I was done with that, I finally asked myself, was my friend right? And the answer was yes. She was right; I am certainly judgmental towards some people. Furthermore, there are some people towards whom I am very judgmental. Simply put, I am not all-loving and poetic all the time.

One such occasion happened on a night when the mother giving birth said the phrase, "I can't take it" about five hundred times straight, like some sort of mantra. After the two hundredth time, I told myself that *I* couldn't take it. In addition, the anesthesiologist stopped her epidural before she was ready for it, and the woman said she felt that she really could not do it without an epidural. After several attempts to cheer her up, to encourage her ("You *can* take it, you're doing great, tell yourself you can...") and at least another ten different tactics (to explain, persuade, accommodate, ask, beg, threaten, shout and ignore her), we called a doctor and asked her to shout at the woman a little, because she claimed she had had enough, could not take it anymore and wanted the baby to be delivered by Caesarean.

So the doctor came, yelled at her a bit, and the woman gave birth in two minutes. Yes, just like that. I judged that woman so much, and I judged myself for judging her and for calling the doctor and actually asking her to yell at that woman.

Another story is the one about *that* father. When I showed him his newborn daughter, he looked at her, said "Great" and continued to walk away and talk on his phone as if nothing had happened. Ugh, I was so angry at him. Or those parents who took pictures of the baby right as she came out, and then dedicated several minutes to admire the pictures, totally forgetting about the living, breathing newborn lying on the mother's belly. I thought they were really strange.

The truth is…it's all true. I sometimes get upset at doctors, and judge other midwives harshly, and get angry at family members, and even at myself. This is how I am. And sometimes it's not anger but just frustration; frustration at people's ignorance; frustration at my own lack of experience and expertise; frustration at situations that I know could be different; frustration at the fact that John Lennon never managed to change the world… and neither have I; frustration at the system and frustration at the times in which we are living. My judgment is not always directed at people, because I am part of that situation too, although it can definitely sound like it at times.

But actually, what am I, if not human? I am not perfect. And good luck about that too! If I was perfect I would be Julia Roberts, and then there would really be nothing left for me to do. Besides, did I mention that I am really fat? For years I have failed at every diet I've tried. Oh dear, what confessions I'm making here.

So, my dear friend, you are on to me. I'm not being sarcastic; it is the truth and I admit it. I am still judgmental, which, by the way, I am trying (and hoping) to stop, or at least reduce. I try to talk with myself and explain the types of behaviors I encounter. I try not to take part in gossip about our patients. I don't express my opinion publicly about what people do. For instance, during the incident with the photograph, I didn't tell that couple to stop this nonsense and look at the baby; I even smiled when they showed me the picture. My goal is to see these women as they are, without judgment, no matter what their choices are and whether I agree with them or not.

By the way, those who knew me at the age of sixteen can testify that I was absolutely intolerable, extremely cynical and very judgmental. Those who knew me at eighteen will say I was even worse. I hope that in thirty years, when I retire, I can look back and say, "Dana, have you noticed how your judgmental attitude diminished over the years? Have you noticed how much unconditional love you have for other people?"

Just one thing -- there are situations in which I don't intend to be tolerant and loving. There are situations toward which I have a very clear stance. Call it being judgmental or whatever you like, I don't care; for example, when a man hits his wife for having a girl instead of a boy. I don't care what the cultural background that made him act this way is, I don't care one bit.

Ahh! I performed an episiotomy -- twice

One of the things that midwives should know is how to make an incision at the entrance to the vagina (an episiotomy[11]). Until I

---

11 A few words about tears and cuts. The original aims of the incision (episiotomy) were: A. To prevent uncontrolled tears. B. To prevent pressure on the baby's head (preterm infants are more vulnerable to the risk of brain bleeding). C. To speed up delivery. There are two types of incision – medio-lateral and midline episiotomy. The medio-lateral one hurts more, bleeds more and heals slower. The midline episiotomy heals quicker and is much less painful, but it is a major risk factor in high-grade tears (including a tear of the anus itself, with all that entails). Therefore, in Israel we do not perform the midline cut, but only the medio-lateral one. For several decades, episiotomies were done frequently during births and still are (in approximately 35% of births in Israel, for example), without any scientific basis that it fulfills the purposes mentioned before. In recent years, methodical research was done on the subject, which found that (surprisingly):

1. The incision does not prevent tears. On the contrary, there are a lot of women whose perineum would stay intact, without rupture or tear, if they were not cut. Beyond that, midline episiotomy represents a significant risk factor for tears in the anus. One study I read had sixty-four cases of rectal tears, of which sixty-three underwent a midline episiotomy. There are many cases of women who suffered tears despite the incision and many more cases in which the incision itself was torn.
2. Tears are divided into four degrees of severity. The incision is like a second degree tear (i.e., both skin and muscle). Some tears (usually first degree tears) do not even require stitching. Of course there may be wider tears.
3. Complications from episiotomy may include pain, infection, loss of blood, damage to pelvic floor muscles, discomfort during sexual intercourse, aesthetic injury, implications for the woman's self-esteem and more.

performed one myself, every time I saw it done I had the chills and felt sick. I really did not understand how I could do it. But, it turns out that, like many things, when the moment of truth comes, it is less terrible than it looks (or at least not that terrible for me. I cannot imagine it being too nice for the mother in question).

The first time I didn't think it was necessary to make the incision, but the unfortunate woman fell under the procedural definition of a patient who must undergo this incision; she had a large baby and this was her first birth. The incision I made was quite tiny (which I admit it was not intentional; I was just a little bit afraid to make the cut), and the baby came out. I called the doctor to sew it up and he was angry that the incision was so small. She needed only two stitches and it probably made him nervous. Idiot! The second time, it seems there was a real need for the episiotomy, because the patient had already undergone three episiotomies in the past

4. The incision does not prevent damage to the baby's head.
5. The incision indeed speeds up the delivery, when it is done at the appropriate time.

One of the reasons doctors prefer an incision over a tear is that it is easier to stitch an incision than a tear, and here again is the discussion regarding the caregiver's comfort versus the patient's. In contrast, the muscle gets torn more naturally and along the muscle fibers, in the case of a tear and not an incision. The new protocol regarding incisions states that they should not be done automatically, but only to speed up the delivery; for example, in cases of fetal distress or when there is a risk of a big tear. Some advocate making an incision in each case of assisted birth, but there are times that this is not required. And we didn't even talk about the dark and mysterious aspects of why men have invented methods of cutting female genitalia (did someone mention female circumcision?). And why they think that our bodies cannot give birth without a pair of scissors. However, it is important to note that there are cases where women tear significantly and as a result, lose control of their sphincters. This just reinforces the point that sometimes an incision is certainly merited, but one should closely examine the cases in which it is absolutely essential.

and a moment before the baby came out she literally almost tore in several places.

Still, I do not like the idea of cutting the perineum. I do not believe in it as a routine work method, and it's hard to tell to what extent the incision is really needed, what is best for the woman, what is best for her perineum, what is best for her pelvic floor and what is best for the baby. I have read quite a few articles on the subject, but experience lends its own weight and importance to the subject. Anyway, I hope I will not have to repeat this procedure too many times.

Of course, there is the matter of the doctors' response to this procedure. I have been at births in which I did not perform an episiotomy and there was a really tiny tear, which needed only a stitch or two or even none at all, and still some doctors were very angry about the fact that I did not perform an episiotomy. Surely a small tear is far better than an incision, except from the perspective that it is a little more complex to sew a tear than a straight cut; but that is the doctor's problem, not the woman's. This is just infuriating and frustrating. When I set up my own maternity ward, there will be none of this nonsense…

And if we are on the subject of tears and cuts, this week I dealt with a woman who had a tiny tear, but would not have any male doctor come within a distance of five meters of her perineum. As there was no female doctor around, all the midwives and me, the intern, consulted, and decided that there was no need for stitches. Later, a female doctor did arrive to check her and said that she believed, for aesthetic reasons, that there was a need for one stitch, but the woman refused, to the delight of all the midwives. By the way, I have read several studies that show that small-to-medium tears heal better when they are not stitched.

What else happened? Well, tonight one of the midwives suggested that I deliver a woman on her side. I was very happy because I had not had the chance to do that so far, because of the reluctance of the women in labor or the instructors who were with me. At first the woman did not want to, but then she agreed to try and found the position very comfortable, so that for most of her contractions she was on her side. At one point, we saw that something was stuck and we advised her to lie on her back again and she gave birth that way. And I must say I was relieved – because the side position is really not a comfortable one for the midwife.

Hold up, hold up. Don't get mad at me. I know that the most important thing is the comfort of the mother and not that of the midwife. I follow this motto on many occasions. On the other hand, I had terrible back pain in the days following this shift and during the delivery. I discussed this with Na'ama, who told me that her back was bad once for an entire month after she supervised a birth where the woman was lying on her side.

So what to do? How to approach this subject? After all, if my back is bad, it will be very difficult for me to deliver, or I would not be able to do so at all, at least for a while. On the other hand, births in different positions have advantages beyond convenience, in terms of tears, speed of delivery, fewer cases of shoulder dystocia, preventing damage to the mother's pelvic floor, etc. So if it's the mother's pelvis versus the midwife's back, which one wins?

I know that if a woman gives birth naturally, say, at home or in water, the midwife does not really have to bend over and take the baby out: the mother does everything by herself. I also know that when you don't tell the mother when to push, especially when you do not shout at her, the baby comes out gradually and slowly, and then you do not need the midwife to protect the perineum. So really, in a natural birth, in all aspects, this would be fine. But what about in a hospital birth, when a woman lies on a bed?

I have to think about something that will help keep my back in shape. Maybe some exercises or perhaps more experience in delivering in unconventional poses.

And one more thing: this week I reached thirty births. There was one shift in which I delivered four women. It was both very exciting and very exhausting. However, it seems to me a bit surreal. After all, every birth is a unique event for the woman, her partner, her baby and the world, if you think about it. To me, it felt completely crazy to run between four such cosmic events within eight hours. At the end of the day, I sat down and tried to remember all the details: the names of the women, what they looked like, what their husbands looked like and what had happened at each birth. Which baby had an umbilical cord around the neck, for which one did I perform an episiotomy and who had a boy or a girl. It was not easy, but I finally succeeded, or at least I think I did.

I understand the economic considerations that prevent allocating a midwife for every woman or two women, and I must admit that not every shift has that many births, and yet, this is not how it supposed to be.

Who cares what I think?

She is having a hard time deciding whether to have an epidural, so she asks me, "What would you do?"

My answer is irrelevant. First of all, because I have never experienced the pain of birth, and second, because even if I had, I had not experienced *her* pain.

"We are two completely different people," I try explaining to her. "What suits me may not suit you." But my answer does not really cut it. It would have been much easier to simply say, "Have an epidural!" or "Don't have one!" - to convince her to give birth the way *I* think is right, to make her want what I want.

One midwife told me she believes that our job is to convince women to have a natural birth. I do not think that my role in the delivery room is to convince anyone to do anything. Why do I need to bring *myself* to the delivery room? Who cares about *my* aspirations, *my* preferences or *my* opinions?

My role in this large theater production called childbirth, at least as I see it, is not the main one. I'm neither the director nor the producer. I have at most a minor role, while at least, I'm just an extra; or perhaps I'm the costume assistant, dressing and undressing the leading actress.

The leading actress in every birth is the mother herself, with her baby showing up for a cameo during the last act. My job, among other things, is to give each woman the required information that can help her make the decisions that work for her.

I realize of course that I cannot teach and tell her everything there is to know during the little time we have together. When a woman asks me, during the brief interludes between her contractions, whether she should have an epidural or some other sedative, and she has no knowledge of the subject, it is clear that any information I give her will be partial or biased in one direction or another. In these situations, I sometimes get the urge to ask, why didn't you take a prenatal course to help you make a more educated choice? But even this question, and the judgmental attitude which it holds, are not included in my job description, so I do not ask. What I am left with is trying to create for every birthing woman the environment that supports and suits her best.

Delivery room or battlefield?

When we arrive for our shift in the morning, there is only one mother in the delivery room; she is in full dilation, without analgesia (she used some laughing gas[12], which doesn't really count). I go to assist her birth and quickly find myself on a battleground.

The mother, screaming and raging, biting herself and her husband, throws herself at the medical equipment around the bed, hurling her pillows everywhere. The husband is a little bit in shock, holding on bravely through this outburst and holding his wife's hand lovingly. The doctor is hysterical because the FHR (fetal heart rate) on the monitor does not look good, and he shouts at the woman to calm down. In response, she gets even more outraged. And I, in my innocence, trying to catch her attention, touch her, while speaking quietly, and get a kick and a strong yank on my hospital scrubs for my efforts.

And it goes on like this. More and more people enter the room, which is not very calming as we all know, until finally, besides the woman giving birth, there are three doctors, three midwives, one husband and one mother-in-law. Everyone is screaming at everyone. The woman kicks the doctor, who in response hits her back on the legs and tells her to spread them already. The woman wants her

12 Laughing gas, or Nitrous Oxide by its scientific name, is used for pain relief in various situations, such as dental treatment. It can be used during birth, but only for limited periods and not for long hours. It causes slight drowsiness, but its effects end quickly after its use stops. Many women find that using laughing gas helps them, while others get discouraged very quickly. Laughing gas does not affect the baby or the birth process.

legs to stay closed, the doctor wants them spread, and there is a small argument about the issue. A urinary catheter is put in with a few more kicks, some yelling, a bit of dissection, pushing and jumping on her belly, the mother-in-law is escorted out, and whoops, the baby is out, congratulations.

I was just appalled at that brutal birth; I did not know under what rock to crawl. I wanted to say in the middle of it all, "I really need to go to the bathroom," and run away, but I stayed. When it was all over, Na'ama asked me cynically, "have you ever heard of a non-violent birth?"

What can be done to prevent this situation? After all, this raging storm began before we even turned up for our shift. How does one maneuver in this kind of chaos, when there isn't any time to talk calmly with the mother, not even for two minutes, because we are having fetal distress, and, in fact, also maternal distress (not to mention delivery room staff distress) ... Ugh!

And why, explain to me why, did the midwife at reception have to give a woman who had just been admitted to give birth, and who was already quite worked up and worried, a five-minute lecture about the importance of bringing her Well Baby Clinic card to the delivery room? Why did this woman have to feel that she had done something wrong from the start?

And why do they tell a woman with twins that it is recommended for her to give birth by Caesarean section, even if the conditions allow for a vaginal delivery? What, just because the doctor doesn't have the nerve for all the hassle that involves the birth of twins?

As you can see, I agree with how the system works every other day. Today was not one of those days.

Push, push, push!!!

A woman giving birth for the first time is in the delivery room. When I arrive for my shift, I am told that she has just been examined and shows a dilation of 6 centimeters. We introduce ourselves. I read her medical record and tell her that if she feels pressure she should tell me. After a minute, she tells me that she feels the need to push. I examine her and ask her what she wants her dilation to be and she says, "Full!" So I reply with a smile, "You've got your wish!"

I suggest she change position according to what she feels is most comfortable, and indeed she decides to lie on her side, and then stand on her hands and knees, and then on her side again, and on her other side. I never instruct her when to push, but she does it all by herself when she feels the need.

By the way, this is something I've been practicing, to stop giving instructions to a woman regarding when to push. After all, this pushing is a natural act that the body does, and just as a woman doesn't need help knowing when to push when she is on the toilet, or need help knowing when to take her next breath, I believe the same applies when she is giving birth. When a woman has been given an epidural, it is a different story. She usually does not feel the pressure or cannot control her muscles properly. In those cases, guidance is needed.

It's not that simple for me not to instruct a woman when to push, since the overwhelming majority of midwives do "push" women - this is how it's referred to in obstetrics lingo - and I hear a lot of "Push, push, push!!!" in the delivery room. If I do not shout like they do, then they tell me I'm not assertive enough.

They do not understand that I just do not want to yell at the women. I believe that women can give birth without someone shouting at them. What? Zebras are unable to give birth without a midwife zebra neighing "*Push, push*" at them?

Anyway, she pushes when she feels it is necessary, and soon the baby's head descends and crowns. My instructor today is Debby, a lovely midwife with whom I have not had the chance to work with before, and she accepts and even encourages all my crazy ideas, such as having dim lights or that we don't automatically result to using an incision. Finally, the baby emerges, the whole process having been nice and smooth. There is a small tear that gets sewn with a couple of stitches and the mother nurses the baby for an hour. He just did not want to leave her breast.

Just before we transfer her to the maternity ward, a woman giving birth to her sixth child comes in with a dilation of 8 centimeters. At a sixth birth, an 8-centimeter dilation is usually very close to ten. It can take just a few seconds to reach full dilation. She went into the delivery room, a beautiful woman with chocolate skin and big sad eyes. My wonderful instructor told me, "Let's give her a natural birth. We won't put an intravenous drip, we will turn off the lights and we won't take apart the bottom section of the bed. In short, we won't do anything." And so we did. Well, I mean, we didn't.

Within fifteen minutes, her baby girl was already out, beautiful just like her mother. I placed her on her mother's belly and waited for the umbilical pulse to stop[13]. Debby was excited and said, "Did

13 A few words about cutting the umbilical cord. After the baby's birth, a significant portion of its blood, up to one third, is still in the placenta and the blood vessels that lead to it. Immediate cutting of the cord prevents the blood from returning to the baby's body. Many studies have shown that an immediate clamping of the umbilical cord leads to an increase in cases of anemia until the age of six months. In most cases, there is no immediate need to cut the umbilical cord and it is possible to wait a few minutes until the pulse in

you see? Did you see?" Even the doctor who wrote the birth summary (the same doctor who once asked a woman, "What is this nonsense I hear about natural birth? Is there such a thing? What are you, a giraffe?") said, "The next time she could give birth at home, am I right?"

---

the umbilical cord stops naturally. In addition, late clamping allows the baby to start breathing gradually rather than having to breathe spontaneously at once, as he continues to receive oxygenated blood from the placenta during the first minutes of his life. When you want to save the cord blood for the purpose of stem cell production, the clamping of the umbilical cord will be performed immediately after delivery or a few minutes later.

The hidden cry

Speaking of this doctor, Dr. Taciturn (a pseudonym)... At first, I thought he was one of the most unfriendly doctors I had ever met; a stoic person who wouldn't utter a single redundant word. If you ask him a question, he just growls something back, never smiling, never even angry; sluggish and apathetic. Once he came into a delivery room that was lit at the time with a lovely dim light, which gave it a special atmosphere, and wham - he turned all the lights on, even without really needing them. The husband asked him politely to turn off the lights and he responded loudly, "Excuse me?" So the husband went over and turned off the lights himself, which really shocked Dr. Taciturn.

Anyway, until last week I never managed to connect with him. He would ignore any question asked by me or the couple; I even saw him once checking a woman who was screaming in pain during the procedure, and heard him say, "What are you screaming about? This doesn't even hurt you!"

So what happened last week? I decided it was time to start communicating with him, to give us a chance at improving our relationship. And as often occurs, when one makes a firm decision, the impossible happens. For starters, I tried telling a few jokes and being a little more open-minded about his methods. Almost immediately, something changed. It's not that he became Dr. Nice all of a sudden, absolutely not, but a new channel of communication opened up, and there was more progress on this front every day. The next milestone was when he critiqued the way I had washed one of the women after birth. It was a correct observation, and I realized that he wanted me to give professional care to our patients, so I thanked him. Later, he gave me a compliment about something I had done, and I thanked him again. Seeing him softening a bit around the edges, the next day I asked him to teach me how to rupture the amniotic membranes, which is a medical procedure at this hospital and not usually performed by the midwives. He agreed and taught me patiently and thoroughly, with all the little details that make this procedure more than just something technical, and providing me with the reasoning behind every step. From there on, the path to open smiles and affection shortened.

I remind myself that everyone has his own hidden tears, the cry that he or she never utters out loud. Our behavior often tries to disguise these tears, but if you scratch the surface a little and wait, without judgment but rather with love, you can sometimes find the person behind the mask. I do not know what the hidden tears of Dr. Taciturn are. Maybe something in his personal life; perhaps his professional career was full of hardship; maybe he does not like the system and tries to survive in it, just like me? I just know he's exceptionally professional at what he does and that the wellbeing of the mother and baby are of the utmost importance to him. I also know that he is not inclined to be influenced by what people think of him and how other people want him to be, and that this is a rare quality. Now that I think about it, maybe I'll call him Dr. Likable.

Three birth stories: the first a little sad, the second a little unpleasant, and the third a bit frustrating

A few days ago, I attended the birth of an Ethiopian immigrant. She arrived in Israel only a year ago and still does not speak Hebrew. Fortunately, there was a sweet national service volunteer with us who could translate. I kept telling her, "Hey, you two look so much alike," and as it turned out, they really were relatives - their grandparents are siblings.

I was a little sad to think that this woman had given birth to four children in a hut in Ethiopia, in her natural environment, surrounded by her family, without ever having a vaginal exam; while here, in Israel, in the Holy Land, she had to lie alone in bed, connected to a monitor and an IV, wearing a standard hospital robe and getting ready to have her baby while lying on her back.

I asked her what position she had been in when she gave birth in Ethiopia, but she was ashamed to say. I demonstrated various positions, of squatting, bending, standing and what not, but she just looked down, which is a sign of respect, and murmured that she would give birth in bed. Finally, she dared to say that what she really wanted was to give birth on her side. I had to leave her quite early, but I made the national service volunteer swear to stay by her side until the end. It was so sad how this woman felt that her way, the way she had always given birth before, was wrong or not good enough. Incidentally, this is also true for breastfeeding, in Ethiopian women. Many of them, who used to nurse their babies for long periods of time, don't do that anymore, because they believe it will not be looked upon favorably in Israel. Why is it that aggressive cultures eradicate subtle and natural ones?

The next day, I asked about her, and as it turns out in the end she gave birth on her back with her legs up, just like everyone else. What can you do? That's just the way things are.

Yesterday, a woman arrived at reception fully dilated. Within a few minutes, she felt the need to push, and everyone got a bit nervous, because the weight estimate suggested a large baby and it was unknown whether she had previously had a problem with shoulder dystocia. Despite continued worries, the birth proceeded in its natural course, and just as the head of the baby was sticking out, there was a power outage in the delivery room. This was not one of those split-second power outs we sometimes have every Tuesday at 7:30 sharp, when they check the hospital's generators, but a long one of at least half a minute or so. For a moment, we were in pitch blackness, since there are no windows in the delivery room. We had no choice but to continue in these conditions, and to tell the truth? It turns out that you don't have to see in order to deliver a baby, and certainly not in order to have one. So the head came out, and then the shoulders, and then the rest of the body happily followed.

After the baby came out (and indeed it was really big -- over eight pounds), the lights turned back on, so I looked at the vaginal opening and waited for the placenta to be expelled. I told myself I'd never seen such a birth, without a single drop of blood, just a shiny umbilical cord dangling down. And as soon as this thought crossed my mind, I touched the belly to see if the placenta had separated already and... *splaaaash* - a huge squirt of blood spattered on the floor, the walls and on me, of course.

It was a great reminder that you never know what's going to happen, and that every moment holds a surprise for us. The last time this had happened, another midwife had pressed on the belly and

I was standing right in front. Guess what happened to my clothes (including my underwear...).

I'm sorry if this sounds disgusting. I'm actually quite enjoying all of this dealing with blood, amniotic fluids, placentas and the like. I don't know why, although I occasionally do wonder. Maybe it's some sort of Freudian sublimation of murderous tendencies? I don't think so. It is just, well, there is something in it; something primordial, perhaps.

After this blood-soaked birth, I joined a delivery room where a woman was giving birth for the first time. It was a very special experience, but in the end it was very frustrating. This woman was not someone you might call beautiful, not at all. But when I approached her, and at that point I hadn't yet said anything, she grabbed my hand and looked me directly in the eyes, and I felt a feeling which is hard to describe in words, although I can recreate that feeling for myself as I am writing this. It was as if her soul was peering into mine, directly; without any interruptions or mediations of flesh and bone. And something from inside of her called out to something inside of me, with such power, sadness and longing; something that asks a question, something that clings tightly, something innocent, something inner. This is just an attempt, and not a very good one, to try and describe the feeling. This woman shone and glowed and was so beautiful to me. Have you noticed that all pregnant women and mothers are beautiful?

After a few hours, she was fully dilated, but the baby's head had not descended into the birth canal, despite all the pushes, turns, standing on hands and knees, lying on the side, trying to relax and whatnot. It was so frustrating to have arrived at this stage and be unable to move one bit further for over three and a half hours. Dr. Likable said all the time, "Don't worry, she will give birth eventually!" Who would have thought it? Dr. Likable, I thought your line was supposed to be, "Let's give her a vacuum!"

Finally, it was decided that the solution would be a Caesarean section. It was impossible to vacuum the baby's head, since it was so high in the birth canal and it was uncertain if the vacuum would work in such a situation. In the operating room, the doctors checked to see if perhaps the head had descended by now, in which case the woman could deliver, but no. It turned out that the baby was upside down, i.e., with his face up, which is called occipital posterior position. Apparently that's what had prevented him from descending into the pelvis. We had actually tried postures that should have helped in this situation, but to no avail. How frustrating and scary.

After I had brought the baby from surgery, Na'ama said to the father, "The important thing is that now you are a family. And it doesn't matter how it happened." It's a statement that might sound like a cliché, but at that moment, and in the way she said it, it didn't sound cliché at all. Rather, it was heartwarming, and really gave me the feeling of family: Father, mother and baby. Now you're a family. It has such a beautiful ring to it.

Tomorrow I'll go to visit her, the one who peered into my soul.

Timing is everything

There are times when it is really not recommended to come to the delivery room, times when it is really not recommended to give birth.

For example, if you turn up at the delivery room just as we are changing shifts, you will be in for a long wait, as it can take up to half an hour until the new shift starts working. So here's a message for all the pregnant women out there, please memorize this: Do not come to the delivery room at seven in the morning, three in the afternoon or eleven o'clock at night.

It is also not recommended that your birth go on past ten in the evening. At that time, the doctors want to "clear out" the delivery room before they go to sleep, and they perform Caesareans on every birth that gets a bit stuck. If you're struggling with your delivery at eight in the evening, that's fine; we'll give you plenty more time to find your natural course, but the later it gets, the more doctors will tend to cut the procedure short - literally. Though I find it hard to admit, this behavior has a certain kind of logic to it. Would you like your doctor and anesthesiologist to be refreshed and alert, or would you prefer them to be still drowsy after being woken up in the middle of the night?

The use of birth induction drugs is also affected by the time of day. The doctor comes up to you and tells you how important and how critical it is to start labor, because the baby is at risk, the pregnancy is at risk, the placenta has aged, the volume of amniotic fluid is low and what have you. You start to worry and get anxious and wish you could get this over with, and then you realize that it is now eight o'clock in the evening and dispensing of birth induction drugs will only resume tomorrow at eight in the morning. This is a really urgent matter, apparently.

Finally, if you do not want to give birth by Caesarean section, do not come for a routine checkup at the end of the month. I swear I'm not making this up, but one day during my internship, which just so happened to be the 30th of the month, the number of births that month had almost reached three hundred. Everyone wanted it to go over three hundred, because then they would get more funding or more staff or who knows what. But they were a few births short of that target, so every woman who came to the delivery room immediately received a tempting offer for induction or Caesarean section. After all, the most important thing was to reach three hundred births.

I know there are financial considerations, I know there are staffing considerations and I know some of it is done for the wellbeing of the mothers, and that it's not a bad thing to take care of the staff's wellbeing as well. And still, isn't a woman entitled to the same quality of care, regardless of the time of day or the day of the month in which she is admitted? Or at least, isn't she entitled to know the considerations involved?

Honest disclosure: I have a very negative opinion of the nursery

As a nursing student, when I worked in the nursery, I burst into tears after ten minutes and it took me an hour to calm down afterwards. I cried because of some mean comments made by the head nurse, and probably due to my hypersensitivity, but after that, it was hard for me to really enjoy working there and I slipped out of it whenever I could. As a nurse in the maternity ward, I go into the nursery almost every day now, sometimes more than once, but I still try to get out of there as fast as I can.

As a midwifery student, this is the third nursery I have had dealings with. It's the nicest of the three by far, as nice as a nursery can be, that is. First of all, it's very small and there is no room for all the babies, so most of them are rooming-in, partly or fully. In other words, they are with their mothers for most of the day and sometimes at night too. The staff members are very pro rooming-in and do everything they can to help the women. They also encourage breastfeeding. Overall, relatively speaking, and I emphasize the "relatively," this place is okay. And yet...

Most of the time, babies in the nursery cry, and I cannot take it. You must understand, it's not that one baby is crying, but ten, and everyone ignores them. At first, I tried to run from one to the other, picking them up, calming them down and singing to them. But after you put them back down, they start crying again; apparently they want their mothers.

When I mentioned that I was finding it difficult to ignore their cries, the nurses said, "Don't be silly! You'll get used to it within a few days." Who would want to get used to it? If I were to get used to ignoring crying babies, how would it affect me? I know that nurses who work there do not want to ignore the babies, they simply have no choice, because there are lots of babies and only two nurses, and they need to weigh, bathe, change diapers, feed and care for all of them. There is no way they could do it if they had to devote their full attention to every baby.

The doctor tells every woman during his round that she should "add a bottle of formula to the baby's diet." Why? Why have such a light hand on the trigger? How can it be that all babies need extra formula? What, none of the babies would be fine with only their mother's milk? The balance of milk production in early lactation is so delicate that any intervention might harm it, sometimes irreparably. It is certainly true that some babies need the extra nutrition from formula, but surely not all. And this is from a hospital that declares itself to be pro-breastfeeding.

One mother asked the doctor what weight her child should be before they discharge him (I must say that even the usage of 'they' and 'discharge' infuriate me. After all, the baby is hers, as well as her responsibility, and it is her right to take him home whenever she wants to. Of course it is recommended she do so after she gets an explanation from the doctor about his condition and what the recommended treatment is. This may sound trivial, but the language we use shapes our ways of thinking. So many times I've heard women ask, "May I get out of bed?" or "Can you let me hold the baby?" like they have no say in these decisions.) The doctor replied angrily, "It's none of your business. We are doing tests. You continue to breastfeed him and give a formula bottle of course, and we will tell you when he can go home."

During the morning examination, the doctor strips every baby in a cold and methodical way, examines it, touches the baby's backside and then leaves him naked for the mother to wrap it up again. And then - without washing his hands – he moves on to the next baby. It goes on like this with all twenty babies. Later, they wonder how infections are transmitted in the nursery. After the end of the visit, I talked about it with my instructor. She said she would talk to him about it, but she almost never washes hands herself, while there.

By the way, that reminds me that a few days ago, during rounds at my hospital, I suggested to one doctor that she disinfect her hands after she touched a patient's infected surgical wound. She told me: "Dana, you really are suggesting the right thing, you really, really are. But this disinfectant gives me a rash so I'd better not." I suggested she use gloves, although it does not really reduce the need for hand washing, but she said there was no need for that. And hand washing is out of the question all together. It takes too long to wash your hands...

And so it goes. It turns out that for many people, Louis Pasteur's germ theory of diseases is still a theory. I think the main problem is that you cannot see germs with the naked eye, and despite all the "progress" of the human race, we still rely mostly on what we can see. It would be obvious to a doctor with blood or pus on his hands that he should wash them, mostly because it is visible. Besides, you must understand doctors. They are dealing with matters far more important than hand washing! They are healers, surgeons, diagnosticians; they prescribe medications and expensive CT scans!

Eitan is always saying, "Most people are like sheep," and unfortunately, it is sometimes true. People just do not think. Do you really think that back in the days of Semmelweis people did not realize that it was unhealthy to go straight to the delivery room with dirty hands after performing an autopsy? If they didn't realize, then they must have been a bit stupid, and if they did realize and carried on regardless, then they really *were* stupid.

There are very few physicians who wash their hands properly, and I really appreciate the ones who do. Unfortunately, I too am still not one of those who wash their hands *properly*, which means to wash your hands for fifteen seconds with soap and water after coming into contact with anything. For example, if I accidently touched the blanket of a patient, I would have to wash my hands.

But after all, believe it or not, it was relatively okay in the nursery. The staff was nice to the families, helping and guiding them. Not too many unnecessary tests and treatments were performed, and most babies were with their mothers, and this is perhaps the most important thing of all.

I have always loved hearing and reading stories about births

Ever since I was a child, I have been captivated by the stories of my grandmother, who told us hundreds of times about how she got to the delivery room reception, how she said goodbye to my grandfather and how the baby came out before he could exit the hospital. I didn't mind that the story never changed, and that the tone in which my grandmother spoke always stayed the same. I always held my breath at the same points, and always felt relieved at the same points. My mother's birth stories and, in recent years, those of my mother-in-law, I obviously know by heart, and never tire of hearing them.

Actually that's what made me want to become a midwife. I realized I felt a calling for the field after understanding that I could hear a million stories and never tire of them. And now, these stories are part of my life too, and I am part of the lives of so many others.

Today, for example, I assisted at three births. The first was a quick one - probably someone with the same genetics as my grandmother; the second was completely natural, which caused the midwife, meaning me, to be a bit battered and bruised at the end of the birth (try chasing a rampant perineum and you'll understand why...) and the third was challenging: a woman giving birth for the first time to a baby weighing almost nine pounds. Nobody believed she could give birth, including me. She lay for hours with pethidine, then an epidural, and nothing happened; the baby's head did not descend into the birth canal. They shaved her pubic area in preparation for a Caesarean section and took the appropriate blood tests, and all the time, doctor after doctor would enter the room, stare at the monitor, which looked terrible, with lots of fetal pulse decelerations, sigh, shake their heads and leave.

Upon arriving at this third and final birth for the day, I went immediately to the mother's side, and was sorry to discover that I too had the uneasy feeling that there was no other option but to resort to Caesarean section. But both of her mothers - I mean her mother and her mother-in-law - were so positive, giving no thought of resorting to surgery, that their optimism was contagious. We joked and sang a little bit to the rhythm of the fetal heart, which was tricky, since it changed all the time. Then we did a little dance and were all in good spirits.

The mother said she did not know how she could give birth to such a large baby, so I told her, "you are a big lady and you'll give birth to a big baby. I don't see any problem with it." Eventually she started to push, and slowly the head descended.

The frustrating thing was that whenever the doctor came into the room, the woman was in between contractions and the monitor didn't show anything. So every time he would say, "The head hasn't come down yet, eh?" and then the moment he left the room, she would start pushing and the baby's head would pop out from her vagina.

A short time after - half an hour in total, which is very nice for someone giving birth for the first time - she gave birth, with a really small incision, to a big, beautiful baby girl with an umbilical cord wrapped around her neck which was probably why the monitor had showed pulse decelerations. The baby sucked happily on her mother's breast, totally clueless that everyone had been predicting she would be born by Caesarean section.

On the one hand, I was very happy and proud that this is how things ended, and felt I had played a part in it. But on the other hand, I too had been questioning her ability to give birth to the baby. I had followed the herd. I even told the anesthesiologist, when I invited him to give the epidural, that she would most likely give birth by Caesarean section.

This should teach me a lesson about believing in maternity, childbirth and the natural wisdom of the body. In most cases, God does not put eight pound babies into women who cannot give birth to them, which is something that I must not forget.

When you're not alone

I don't like the phrase, "I've delivered a baby." It's as if the woman didn't do this all by herself but *I* did it for her. In the ward, we say, "I attended a birth," and I like it. Anyway, yesterday I attended two births. The first was short and simple – the birth of a fifth child, which took place fifteen minutes after I met the woman. By the way, I have noticed that a lot of births occur, for some reason, during the first half hour after the shifts change. Maybe it's because the mothers did not connect with their previous midwife, and then after her shift ends and a new midwife arrives, they feel different and give birth? Interesting, isn't it? Maybe the opposite is also true: a woman is about to give birth and 'bam' the shift ends, and they get stuck for hours?

The second birth was a real joy. This was a woman giving birth for the first time, an ultra-Orthodox woman who came with her husband, mother and a wonderful doula,[14] who used to be a home birth midwife back in the US. She chose not to take out a license here in Israel, as it turns out that it's a complicated process, and so she just works as a doula instead. Some midwives turn up their noses at women who come to the delivery room with a doula, but not all of them, certainly not all of them. Now, after I attended for the first time the birth of a woman who came with a doula, I still wonder what I think about it.

---

14 A doula is a birthing assistant, a woman who provides counseling, support, encouragement and assistance to women during different stages of pregnancy, birth and early parenthood.

First of all, it was great that she had a doula with her, because her husband was out of the room most of the time and despite that, the woman had great support throughout her birth. The two women embraced and encouraged her, and even when I could not be in the room, because I had to take care of other women as well, I knew she was not left alone.

The doula gave massages with scented oils, encouraged the woman to move more, and convinced her that she should go into the hot tub: all things I had already offered her, but which most mothers shy away from or are not interested in and the subject never comes up again. In this case, the doula probably told her about all these possibilities in advance, and the mother wanted to experiment. This way, we passed the time, six hours or so, until we achieved full dilation, without using any analgesic medication, and it was great. The mother was charming, and in between contractions she was either smiling or sleeping.

But later, the doula convinced the mother to ask for an amniotomy that she did not need; she convinced the woman to have an enema, although she was quite hesitant about it; she told her to push the instant she reached full dilation, even though she did not feel the urge to push; and she explained how to push in the exact opposite manner to what is recommended if you want to maintain a healthy pelvic floor: "Keep your mouth closed, do not exhale, push down with all your strength, hold the bed handles..."

At this point, I did not know what to do. On the one hand, it's true that the woman chose the doula to accompany her during the birth, and she had left me little choice. But does this mean that when a doula is present, I should deal solely with medical issues and not interfere in matters that are not purely medical? On the other hand, I was still the midwife at this birth and I too am allowed to explain, recommend or advise things – even things that might contradict the doula's advice. But then again, the sense of security and trust in the people around you when you are giving birth is very important. At that time, it's probably not appropriate for the midwife and doula to have a debate over your head while you're panting and pushing. Contradictory instructions are also not a good idea, neither is a sense of suppressed hostility. Now don't get me wrong, there was no hostility at all; we had fun together. I'm just trying to learn from the situation.

In the end, everything was fine and I would love to work again with this doula. There was great value to her presence, even if there were specific things that struck me as wrong.

One of those things was that after the woman gave birth, the doula and the woman's mother wanted to go home. And right at that point, the delivery room got really busy and crowded and I could not attend to the new mother, and all this was just as she was struggling with breastfeeding. I asked them to stay a little longer, so they stayed a few minutes more. I felt it was more prudent to stay with her at least an hour after the birth, rather than to disappear immediately. On the other hand, it was quite a long birth for them, too, so I understand the difficulty.

During the birth itself, I was confronted with another dilemma, which I haven't resolved yet. The mother told me she had been given a perineal massage[15] during the month prior to birth, and she asked me not to cut her. According to procedure and the evaluation of the fetal weight, which was not particularly high, that was possible. I told her that if I saw we must cut, then we would cut; and if not, we would not. When the baby's head emerged, and it took a few good contractions until it did, it came out a little way and went back again, came out and went back, and it took a few contractions

15 Perineum - the area between the vaginal opening and the anus. Most of tears during childbirth occur in this area and so does the episiotomy. This is also the area that it is recommended to massage towards the last weeks of pregnancy, in order to reduce the chance of tears.

more for the head to get halfway out. Na'ama told me that I should cut the woman so the baby could come out already and to stop her suffering, but I did not want to; the perineum was really flexible and I really hated the thought of just cutting it against the woman's wishes.

I asked Na'ama if she believed the woman's perineum would tear, and she said it would happen for sure. She added, "You know, in these kinds of cases, one is either a man or a mouse." She finally ruled:

"Just cut it already."

I picked up the scissors while my stomach turned, but by then it was too late to cut. The head was past the point of no return and came out. Eventually, the woman had no external tearing, and inside there was only small scratch that needed no stitches. I was so happy I didn't cut her. It's really great to have your first birth without stitches. It probably means that the rest of your births will also be like that. So I guess I turned out to be a man this time.

But wait, what would have happened if I had needed to cut her? What would have happened if the woman tore so badly that they had needed to stitch her under full anesthetic? And what if she had, partially or fully, lost control over her anal muscles, which happens in rare cases?

And from this, a bigger question emerged: whether, in order to prevent serious damage to a very few women, we are allowed to cause slight to moderate damage to most women? And who exactly decides this? Should the woman decide if she takes the risk? Should she be given all the information needed to make the right decision? Should I take the risk instead? Should the doctor? Should the Ministry of Health? What about the fact that the medical system operates today primarily to avoid getting sued? Doctors say, "I don't care that she said she doesn't want us to cut her. What does she know about it? When she tears and loses anal sphincter control for the rest of her life, the court won't care that she did not want us to cut her." How can you work like that? All relevant considerations get tossed to one side.

Another question is, how to take action so that the doctor won't be angry with me? I would have no problem with him being angry, if this had no other implications, such as for example, to what extent will he trust me next time to manage a delivery, and to what extent will he, as a result of his attitude toward me, intervene in my job? Maybe the price of an episiotomy is better than constant interference in a delivery?

There are so many questions on my mind, and I have a feeling they will not soon be answered... the problem is that this is not a philosophical dilemma for me. This is something genuine and real, according to which I will very soon, tomorrow actually, have to act.

In the interim

This week, I finished my first internship. In a week and a half I will start my second internship, at a different hospital this time. In the period between our two internships, we will return to our studies at the midwifery school.

When we caught up again at school, my friends asked me, "Well, how was it?" And when I said it depended, that there were things I enjoyed and things that I really didn't like, most of them glared at me in puzzlement: how can it be that I did not get along wonderfully in my internship? What, you want to tell me it wasn't perfect?!

I imagine that the rest of the students did not enjoy every minute of things either. I think that part of their puzzlement was related to how I expressed myself. Some people, when you ask them how they are doing, will say "Okay," and others will elaborate a bit more. I think that the definition of a bothersome person is someone who really answers when he's asked how he's doing. There is something in us that wants to put everything in a box, cut into cubes, condensed and concise; something that wants life to be as simple as a multiple choice test answer:

How was the experience?

A. Fantastic.
B. Not that great.
C. Bad.
D. Okay.

A more detailed answer is not welcome.

Besides, it seems to me that a lot of things that bug me do not bug the others so much, and maybe because of that they had a more pleasant experience, with a little less self-contradiction and fewer stomach turns. I've always been a bit childish and passionate, taking it all too seriously. Only in recent years have I begun to see that there are many shades of gray and that not everything is black or white.

But me, myself, how do I really feel about my experience? I learned a lot of things, such as how to: perform vaginal examinations (sometimes there were differences between my instructor and me, regarding how dilated the cervix was. For example, I thought a cervix was fully dilated and she thought it was only at 2 centimeters... probably she was right...), admit a woman, make an incision, help the doctor with an epidural, check the placenta, care for the newborn, accompany a Caesarean section, help women during labor, do an enema and install an intravenous drip, find the FHR on the monitor, write a nursing report, clean a room after birth, check whether the uterus has contracted and assess the amount of bleeding after birth, recognize fetal distress on the monitor, induce labor, perform an amniotomy, check to see if the perineum has torn, deliver a woman according to Bratslav *Halacha*, Lithuanian *Halacha*, Chabad *Halacha* and Shas *Halacha*[16], communicate with an Arab woman, deliver a woman who won't say a word...

But more importantly, I've learned how to connect quickly with people, how to handle four women at once and treat them in the correct order of priority, how to work under pressure, how to swallow a slice of bread and cheese and gulp down a cup of coffee in

16 These are all religious groups of ultra-Orthodox Jews in Israel. They all share many beliefs and customs, but can also be extremely different in their ways and behaviors. The Halacha is the collection of their rules, ways and means, religious acts and daily actions, including how to behave when giving birth or when assisting a birthing woman.

under forty-five seconds, how to argue with a doctor diplomatically, how to step aside when the placenta comes out in order to not get blood all over myself, how to deliver a woman who is kicking me, how not to get upset, what is the proper way to get upset, how to relax quickly, how to get others to relax, how to ask for something from the doctor without making her come into the delivery room, how to avoid making a cut, how to postpone inducing labor for as long as possible...

I learned many things I'm happy about, and all the rest I store in a special mental drawer called, "Temporary only, please forget in six months." Then again, there are things I store in a drawer called, "To remember and use for as long as I work in a hospital." It's not easy, but I hope my drawer method succeeds. I think it might work if I put things in the correct mental drawer in advance. It's harder if everything goes into one general drawer, and only later gets sorted out into the things that I want to keep with me for life and the things I prefer to leave behind.

What's the big deal? It's basically just another public hospital

How different could it be? So apparently it can be very different. There are many small differences, mostly for the better. For example, in this delivery room, there is no protocol that states we must make an incision in every woman giving birth for the first time, to a baby over a certain weight; there are no orders that we must perform an episiotomy in certain circumstances; in fact, they leave that decision to the discretion of the person attending the delivery. Today, for example, I saw the head of the department perform a vacuum-assisted delivery without making a cut, which is really rare.

They don't pressure the mother to do an enema and they don't force women to be admitted; although they do try to convince them to be admitted, but that is different from a situation in which women don't even know they have a choice. There is no gossiping about women; they do not cut the cord until after the placenta is delivered; they do not push on the belly to get the placenta out; they do not disassemble the bed before birth; they try to avoid leaving the woman in the hallway after giving birth, while transporting her from the delivery room, as everyone, including the doctors, cares about the mother's privacy; they encourage breastfeeding after birth and that the baby will stay with its mother for prolonged periods; and much more.

The team seems very independent, and there is a good relationship between colleagues, no hostility between doctors and midwives, and fewer commands like, "take her blood tests." I've seen some absolutely fantastic sights, like a doctor looking for an IV stand for a woman so that she could move around. Who ever heard of a doctor doing such a thing? I haven't encountered that in any other department I've worked in. So far, I've only known doctors to shout at nurses, "Bring me an IV stand," but here the doctors are really nice.

On the other hand, there are of course things here that are not as good as the other hospital; such as the fact that mothers are not allowed to eat during labor, and the fact that they check on them every hour (unless the woman refuses, in which case they don't push it too hard). There are probably other things that I just haven't discovered, simply because I'm still at reception and not in the delivery room yet. I'm sure there are good things I've not found out about yet, too. I know, for example, that delivering in various positions is really common here. Overall, it is a great delivery room and I'd love to work here in the future.

My first day was pretty exciting. It started with a shocking vacuum delivery. Actually, from what I've seen so far, all vacuum deliveries are shocking. It was carried out due to fetal distress, and unfortunately my shock showed all over my face. Michal, my new instructor, remarked that I might at least look a little less shocked. But how can you not be shocked when you see an oversized doctor pulling with all his might at a suction cap attached to the top of the baby's head; the same head that later will be caressed by his grandmothers, who will not let any of the family's toddlers touch it because it is so delicate. The baby was born almost dead - he still had a pulse, but he was not breathing - so I witnessed cardiopulmonary resuscitation as well.

After the vacuum delivery ended, they called me to watch a forceps delivery of a tiny premature baby, weighing less than 3 lb, 1 oz. This was also a difficult experience, especially for the mother, who screamed and screamed. I'm getting tears in my eyes now, just from thinking about it. Immediately afterwards, she apologized for shouting so loudly, which made it even sadder. Why should you apologize for shouting, when you are in terrible pain, and without any anesthetic? Why do women think it is expected of them that they be good little girls who are quiet, polite and clean? Why? Maybe because that actually *is* what's expected of us.

It sounds strange; the description of these assisted births,[17] the first ones I experienced in this internship, in comparison to what I said about this delivery room. However I believe it was simply an unhappy coincidence, and in many ways this really is a much better delivery room.

---

17 A few words about assisted deliveries. There are certain situations in which a delivery is completed using a vacuum cup or forceps. Usually this happens in cases where labor is not progressing or if there is fetal distress. For an assisted birth to be carried out, the woman should be fully dilated, and the baby's head must be low enough in the pelvis that it can be grabbed. An episiotomy is performed in most cases, unless this is not a first birth and the doctor feels that the woman can deliver without an incision. The main advantage of assisted deliveries is the speed at which the woman delivers. When deciding to perform a Caesarean section, even in the most urgent cases, it may take fifteen to twenty minutes before the infant is delivered. Assisted delivery, in contrast, will generally be much shorter, and take only a few minutes, and when there is fetal distress, every minute counts. The advantage to a woman is the avoidance of Caesarean section, which despite being very common, holds many risks, including to future pregnancies and births. The disadvantages of assisted deliveries include trauma to the baby's head (although life-threatening trauma is very rare) and the mother's pelvic floor (mainly in forceps delivery). Of the two types of assisted deliveries, vacuum birth is safer for the mother and her baby. Its implementation requires less skill, but also takes longer to perform. Forceps delivery requires a highly-skilled operator on the one hand, but on the other, allows a baby to be extracted very quickly, even in situations where vacuum delivery is inefficient or not possible.

A hard day in my internship, a day when I learned a lot, I'm just not sure what

There are many impressions and experiences that I have still not worked out and organized in my head. It started in the morning. We met a mother giving birth for the first time, who was admitted with increased bleeding, which made us suspect early abruption of the placenta.[18] That suspicion eventually turned out to be correct. So we began the process of inducing labor. She had contractions every two minutes, which lasted for a whole minute, i.e., a minute with contractions, a minute without. The labor progressed very quickly, as is usually the case when there is separation of the placenta, and within a few hours she was fully dilated and pushing.

---

18 A few words about placental abruption: During pregnancy, the placenta sits tight against the walls of the womb. It supplies the fetus with oxygen-rich blood and nutrients and evacuates toxins and waste products from its bloodstream. It is supposed to separate from the uterine wall after birth, usually within a few minutes, and be delivered. In fact, this is the third stage of birth - the birth of the placenta. In relatively rare cases, usually due to various risk factors, the placenta separates before birth. If the separation is substantial or full, it could harm the fetus severely, since its blood supply is drastically impaired now. Even the mother's life may be in danger. Fortunately, it is rare to see a complete separation of the placenta and in most cases it is only a separation of a small portion of it, which does not increase, and the pregnancy can sometimes continue for several weeks more; under strict surveillance of course. When a birth begins with a separation of the placenta, it usually means it will progress very fast, and because of that, vaginal delivery is possible in most cases and there is no need to complete the birth by Caesarean section.

I attended the birth with Katie, one of my instructors, and it was so much fun. Here, you do not have to do an episiotomy, you do not have to disassemble the bed, you do not have to do much of anything, actually – you just simply allow the birth to happen on its own. Katie was just wonderful, and taught me something important: that it's a good idea not to panic, even if the situation is really stressful; an important lesson that I had the chance to implement immediately.

The woman's mother-in-law, who was with her in the delivery room, told me that her mother have given birth to sixteen children at home. She herself gave birth at home to "only" seven children. "In those days," she told us, "there weren't so many problems at birth and we did not need doctors and hospitals, only a midwife."

When we finished with the first delivery, we went to the bathroom, drank a quick cup of coffee, and then proceeded to take care of the second delivery. The woman was fully dilated and the baby's head was very low in the pelvis. This was her first birth. Why can't a woman start at her second birth? Giving birth for the first time is so hard, it's almost like parting the Red Sea. The baby was estimated to be over 9 lb, 8 oz.

The threat of birth by Caesarean section, should the birth not proceed accordingly, floated ominously in the air. Basically, everything was ready for surgery: We had an IV drip and epidural at hand; the woman had already been given the required pre-op medication, etc. But my instructor, Katie, was full of faith and believed that everything would be okay.

And everything really was. It wasn't easy for the woman, but gradually the baby descended into the birth canal. At one point, the doctor came in and asked if we had done an episiotomy, and we said that in due time we would, since giving birth to a large baby can result in a serious rupture. Then, as we said, when the right time came, I made the incision. Within a few blood-soaked contractions, the baby was born, but the woman was still bleeding - from the cut of course.

Then it was time to apply the lesson I had learned earlier that day: How not to run amok screaming, but to focus on what is most important right now. When you are anxious, the difficulty is of course to know what is most important. How to function, as three doctors are yelling orders over my head, such as, "I want a blood count!!! Say it's urgent!!! And call the lab!!! Give her another IV!!! Give her Pitocin[19] in the other hand!!!! What's her pulse now???"

I think I understand now what it feels like to be one of the soldiers you see in those war movies, whose training involves going through an obstacle course while someone is shooting live ammunition over their heads. It's a good thing Katie was beside me and occasionally saying things like, "Don't worry, they're just stressed out, back in the old days they wouldn't make a fuss about it, it is fine ..." And everything really was fine in terms of the bleeding, which stopped soon after. What wasn't fine was the fact that the woman had a tear from her episiotomy to her sphincter, which may harm her ability to control defecation in the future.

This is the first time it happened at a birth I attended and the feeling is really terrible. It feels terrible because this was a birth that was under my responsibility, but even more so because this is really bad for the woman.

The doctors debated whether it would have happened if there had been no episiotomy, or whether the situation would have been even more serious if we had not made the cut and whether the

19 Pitocin is an artificial oxytocin that causes uterine contractions and is used for birth induction. After birth, it is customary to give intramuscular or intravenous Pitocin to help contract the uterus and prevent excessive bleeding after childbirth. Some women choose not to receive the drug but to breastfeed instead, an action that may cause the release of Oxytocin in their bodies naturally.

episiotomy had been long enough. I consoled myself with the fact that Katie and the doctor who attended the birth felt I had performed admirably and that the woman just tore. I asked Katie what would have happened if this woman had given birth at home, and she said, "She would have probably not torn at all." But in truth it is impossible to know.

All this happened just before the end of the shift, but Katie and I stayed for another hour or so to see that this dear woman felt well and that everything was fine. I dragged myself back home and crashed on the bed, almost unable to speak. Only after two and half hours of sleep did I recover a little.

So that was my day, an eventful one without a doubt. I experienced some new situations; worked under pressure; coped with rapid decision-making; and dealt with doctors, prolonged first births, large babies, placental abruption, bleeding after birth, perineal tears and more.

I feel like I need to sleep for two weeks just to process it all.

Just a regular old Friday

It started off with a quiet morning. There were no women in labor in the delivery room and none in reception. So we midwives sat down, drank coffee and ate breakfast. And when you have more than one midwife in a room, what do you think they talk about? Well actually there are two main subjects: deliveries and diets, which apparently are the two most interesting topics in the world (in that order: deliveries and diets). I find that this is one of the most successful ways for us midwives to exchange knowledge. One tells about a delivery where the baby's shoulders refused to come out and what they did to solve the situation, and another tells how an umbilical cord prolapsed and what they did to solve this; there was a lot of knowledge and a lot of experience in one room, and there I was in the middle of all this, thirstily drinking in my coffee and their stories.

After they finished their conversation, I went with my instructor to the maternity ward, where we visited Salima, whom we had all taken care of throughout her frightful pregnancy, which ended with her being admitted to intensive care and having a Caesarean section in week thirty-one. Salima has four daughters. Well, actually, five now. However, her husband would very much like to have a boy. In fact, he married Salima after his first wife gave him only girls. (It's obvious to everyone that he only has X-chromosome sperm, right?)

Salima is relatively old to be giving birth and really not that healthy; she has diabetes, heart disease, obesity and chronic hypertension. Besides that, she has already been through four Caesareans. In her current pregnancy she had a pulmonary embolism and almost didn't make it. Each additional pregnancy will endanger her life, but her husband refuses to consent to tubal ligation; he wants a son.

Salima will not agree to undergo tubal ligation without her husband's consent or without his knowledge. I asked her, "So what will you do, Salima?" And she told me with a mischievous smile, "He just won't get any." But I also saw deep sadness and despair in her eyes.

From there we went to visit Salima's baby in the NICU. She is cute and tiny. Salima had described her as being "the size of a kitten." We also went to see a baby with Down syndrome, who had been born overnight. It is important to learn to recognize all the signs in the delivery room, so Katie told me what they are: typical facial characteristics, a typical line in the palm, thick back of the neck, typical shape of the palm, low muscle tone and more. Usually not all the signs are there; it's enough to find only some. The final diagnosis can only be done by a genetic test, because one baby might have just one sign and still have Down syndrome, while another baby might have five signs but not have the syndrome.

It all made me a little sad. It amazes me that people say to me all the time, "Oh my, what a joyful profession you have." And the more I experience the highs and lows of being a midwife, the more I realize how detached from reality this statement is.

The day wore on, and slowly a few women began to drop by reception to check up on their pregnancies, often because their pregnancy was supposed to be "over" already, at least in their opinion.[20] In the opinion of the fetus, the one who actually matters, they were still quite pregnant.

---

20 Prolonged Pregnancy – The duration of a healthy pregnancy is forty weeks on average. However, a baby is considered "ready" starting in week thirty seven. Of course some women give birth after the estimated date of birth. Most hospitals recommend close follow-up of the pregnancy after week forty, i.e., by monitors, ultrasound and movement count by the mother. From week fort- one, and in some places week forty-two, doctors recommend inducing labor to avoid prolonged pregnancy complications, including high rates of

In between tasks, I noticed a woman who stopped every couple of moments to take a breather. Her name was Nasreen and this was her third birth. She had a dilation of 3-4 centimeters and she was walking around reception, stopping and sighing each time she had a contraction. I did not watch her the whole time, but every time I saw her it seemed that her contractions were stronger; she stopped for longer periods of time and took deeper breaths.

After three quarters of an hour, she asked me to check on her because she wanted to get something for the pain. In all her previous births she had been given painkillers and she just had to have them now. I checked her and found a dilation of 6-7 centimeters. I told her that maybe it is not such a good idea, because it seems she would give birth soon, but she still wanted to have it. After a minute or so, she said she felt the baby coming. I checked her again – a 9 centimeter dilation.

Analgesics were now out of the question, and in a wonderful way the body did its magic and released large amounts of endorphins into her bloodstream. She relaxed and lolled between contractions or just dozed off somewhere and with each contraction she murmured, "I really feel it's coming out!" But the baby was still not out. Towards the end of the delivery, the pulse of the fetus on the monitor began to fall eerily - 80, 70, 60 ... (a normal FHR is 110-160 beats per minute) without recovery between contractions. Usually this means there is something wrong with the umbilical cord - maybe it is wrapped around the baby's neck or tied or pinched somewhere, so I called the doctor. The doctor came and tried to help a little, and after two contractions the pulse recovered. The doctor said everything was fine and that we should just continue. So we continued, and after another two contractions the baby was born in a kind of

---

Meconial Water in birth, a large fetus, which can lead to shoulders dystocia during birth, and a slight increase in intrauterine mortality.

strangely rotated way. He came out with his head to the left, turned up and then down again. Anyway, after the head, the body soon followed, and we found ourselves with a sweet baby on our hands. All in all, it took less than two hours from the beginning of contractions to the time of birth. And, by the way, there was a real tight knot in the umbilical cord. In such cases, I always think we should pray to God and give thanks, because such cases do not always turn out so well.

Meanwhile, in the other room, another birth was on its way. Svetlana was giving birth for the fifth time, and her waters had broken about a day ago. She was being induced, at her request. Grisha, her husband, asked me the million-dollar question:

"When is she going to give birth?"

I can't remember participating in a single delivery where I was not asked this question. And it is so tempting to just randomly throw a time out, say, "In four and a half hours." I always feel like they look at me a bit askance when I say there's no way to tell, it could be as little as five minutes or as long as three weeks. And there really is no way to tell. Every midwife has been surprised so many times, in both directions, so it is rare that someone dares to predict an exact birth time. There is also something good in this; it teaches us humility. It gives us an understanding that we do not comprehend everything and that not everything is in our control.

Anyway, I hoped that Svetlana would deliver in the next few hours and not in three weeks, so that I would be able to attend this birth too. And just as I wished, as I went out of Nasreen's delivery, Svetlana was experiencing strong contractions, but she did not want any analgesia. I ran off to eat a quick lunch, and just as I got back, Grisha found me and said, "She's calling for you." I went to check her: 8 centimeters dilated.

"Well," I say, "let's begin to prepare for the birth." I start to open the birth kit and while I deal with removing bandages from the package, I can hear our lovely Svetlana making a sound that is not of this world; I have no other way to describe it. I have never heard such a voice and it's not like anything you can imagine. I look and see the tip of the baby's head looking back at me. I called my instructor to join me and within a minute and a half, the baby was already being embraced by his mother and father. Grisha cut the umbilical cord; the placenta slipped out; there were no tears and Svetlana took out her breast to feed the hungry baby, who wouldn't leave it for another hour and a half.

Both these births were just simple and great, and again I find myself happy with what I do for a living; thrilled by the beauty of the process; amazed at how I, someone who had difficulty getting to know people quickly, find myself meeting strangers and within minutes am part of one of the most intimate situations in their lives. I can feel the great and special complexity in the relationship between Svetlana and Grisha; the strength of Svetlana's will in light of the hardships she has had in life, most of which I'm not privy to, but still know that they were there; Grisha's cheerfulness; the source of strength I know he is for her; the unspoken concerns and problems of Nasreen, in her daily life with her family, with the strong father she grew up with and her courage to live her life to the fullest. All these feelings come to me like the touch of a butterfly on my shoulder, soft yet still clear and strong. Like intricate strands that intertwine people, creating a texture so delicate that it is invisible, yet stronger than any known fabric.

❖ ❖ ❖

Tomorrow I go to class and hope to learn something new and become wiser, but mainly I want to exchange experiences with my fellow students. In truth, if they were to let us sit together for twelve hours, we would not get bored of telling stories about the births we had seen; about the doctors, instructors, mothers, their families, and all that had happened to us in the past month and a half since we met. But we have only two brief breaks of fifteen minutes, and at the end of the day everyone goes their separate ways, so I find my wishes left unfulfilled.

Woo hoo, I've delivered twins!!!

I've delivered twins! I've delivered twins! Woo hoo, I've delivered twins!! This is the song that plays in my head since this morning. I've delivered twins!!!

When I got to my morning shift, they told me that there was a woman about to deliver twins, and that they were vertex-vertex, meaning that both are with their heads down. This was her third birth; she has two daughters at home, and soon she was to have two sons. I entered the room, introduced myself to the couple, and spent the next two hours mostly in search of a pulse on the monitor; the so-called "wonders" of technology. In between, I also fell in love with this woman, who was just delightful during her birth.

Although she did not take anything for the pain, she just sat in bed, quiet and relaxed, smiling between contractions, occasionally skimming a finger across her husband's cheek, as he gently rubbed her back. She had a kind of calming presence, without saying anything in particular or doing something specific, or perhaps because of it. She did not seem worried that she was about to have twins; she was just in the moment.

Her husband was such a darling; he didn't speak Hebrew very well and when he spoke, his Arabic accent was so thick it was hard to understand him. But he had beautiful, kind eyes, and it was obvious that they really love each other. There was such tenderness between them, and respect and space.

There were special moments in those two hours of searching for a pulse. There was one occasion when I entered the room just as the woman was in the middle of a painful contraction. The woman clung to me and we just hugged. I realized that what she needed at that moment was to put her head on someone's chest. Apparently there is such a need at birth. Sometimes I wish I was a sixty year-old grandmother, with white hair tied in a thick bun of course, and huge breasts; the ultimate maternal figure. Someone who had given birth at least five times and has grandchildren; someone who nursed babies for ages, even other women's babies; someone who can hug women during childbirth and who women want to get hugged by. But I am not yet this grandmother, who undoubtedly I one day will become, and yet this special woman hugged me today and I hugged her.

After two hours, she was fully dilated and with great festivity we moved to the operating room to continue the delivery, just to be on the safe side. This doesn't really inspire a sense of security in you, does it? Just the word "operating" alone is pretty scary for most people. But what can you do, some twin births indeed get complicated and require an emergency Caesarean section at some point.

A few other characters joined us along way: a senior physician, an anesthesiologist, the head nurse and an ultrasound machine. I tried not to be excited at all the high-ranking physicians in the room, and in truth it wasn't that hard, since I was already over-excited as it was. Within a few contractions, the first baby was born amid great fanfare, weighing 5 lb, 8 oz. This was the moment when everyone should have become nervous - what if the cervix closed? What would happen if there was too much bleeding? What if the baby suddenly reversed to a breech position? What if the umbilical cord decided to drop from the vagina? A lot of things could have happened, but none of them did. The second twin was still in its amniotic sack. I wondered if he noticed how roomy it had suddenly become inside the uterus.

It was decided to perform a rupture of the membrane, which was conducted by my instructor. And then, during another contraction, the second twin was born. There was a total of nine minutes between the two births. Wow, how exciting (I've delivered twins!).

And then there was a strange situation where there were two umbilical cords hanging from the vagina and all of us were waiting in tense anticipation to see what will come out next?

First came the first placenta, small and beautiful, wrapped in its amniotic sack. More membranes lingered in the doorway, and the second placenta had started to come out as well. I tried to catch one placenta in each hand so their weight would not cause the membrane to rupture. It was an impossible task and in the end the doctor told me, "Forget about it and just let gravity do its work." Just then, the placentas slid undamaged, straight into the bin under the bed. Michal, my instructor, who must have been a midwife for thirty years, told me that she never saw two separate placentas coming out without being connected. Interesting.

And everyone was so happy: these wonderful parents, the doctor, the anesthesiologist, the midwives, the aunties back at home, the babies and everyone who heard about it, even the ultrasound machine. And me? - *I've delivered twins*!!![21]

---

21 A few words about the birth of twins: Twin births are slightly more complicated than regular births due to the high incidence of breech or transverse lie, the fear of cord prolapse or partial separation of the placenta after the birth of the first twin and more. In principle, there is no reason not to give birth vaginally when the first twin's head is aligned downward (the other can be vertex or breech), and when the weight of the first twin is not significantly lower from the weight of the other. Sometimes, due to complications after the birth of the first twin it is necessary to perform a Caesarean section to deliver the second twin. Nevertheless it is generally recommended to try and start the birth vaginally.

Oh, those magical hours of the night!

It is a bit like stepping into another dimension, another world, where the day-to-day toil has no place and everything gets easier, softer, and parts that grate against each other during the day suddenly seem to fall into place and connect.

I spent the night in the realm of the powerful women of the delivery room. And what a night it was; rich with experiences that could fill several event-packed days in terms of their quantity and intensity.

Let me introduce all the characters. First, we have the senior midwife and my wonderful instructor, Katie - a cheerful Irish lady, big and full of soul. A real vibrant woman who loves life, the women she treats and midwifery as a whole. Next is Michal, my second instructor, also a veteran midwife, with a strong love for natural childbirth and the use of common sense. Olivia, the third midwife, is an amazing woman with a fascinating life story. She came to us from Nigeria, Africa - a real special African lady. And then there is me, the intern. There were also two doctors, the nice kind, who slept through most of the shift.

When we came to start our shift, the delivery room contained one woman who had given birth and another who was about to give birth for the first time, and who was still in her latent phase. Right from the beginning, the overarching theme of this shift was empowerment. Most of us knew the woman who had just given birth, from when she came to the delivery room to monitor her pregnancy: A wonderful and powerful woman who knows what she wants. When we met her that evening, she was lying in a dark room with the baby on her breast, after a prolonged feeding, filled with joy. She did not want to part with the baby, so we did not separate them. After we helped her to clean up a bit and move to a wheelchair, she went proudly to the maternity ward with the baby in her arms. This woman was so beautiful and strong, I felt as if I had entered the realm of the Amazons.

Shortly after we escorted her to the maternity ward, a woman in her thirty-second week came from there with premature contractions. She was screaming and crying loudly. Even though she was given various pain medications, nothing seemed to work. Although she wasn't actually about to deliver, she was having really painful contractions, but without any dilation. I think that mainly she was just frightened.

I talked to her a bit and tried to calm her down. I asked where she was from and what her husband did for a living - all kinds of stupid questions, because when you come down to it, I didn't know what to do in this situation either. And then she told me, as if in response to a question I didn't ask, "You see, I haven't even turned seventeen yet." And it explained a lot about her fear, which intensified the pain so much. In the end, she fell asleep in our ward and spent the night there. I think maybe what she really needed was to have her mother by her side.

After she fell asleep, Michal and I went to introduce ourselves to Yael, the woman who was still in her latent phase. She lay in the room after two days of frequent and painful contractions, and she was completely exhausted. I opened her medical chart and saw that she had a birth plan. Oh dear. Birth plans always scare me a little. Somehow it always turns out the opposite of what was expected. With her were her lovely husband and loving sister, who just so happened to be a yoga instructor for pregnant women.

Yael's journey would be an arduous one and would include many more hours of painful and frequent contractions, an epidural at 5 centimeters ("Bless you, bless you," she would pray over and over to the God of epidurals...), a few more hours stuck with a dilation of 5 centimeters; Pitocin augmentation, which would progress the dilation to 8 centimeters; and fear, one great fear of the threat of a Caesarean section. I do not know how Yael gave birth in the end, but I know she was a real fighter the whole way. She was inhaling and exhaling with each contraction, mumbling something in a low voice to her husband, turning from side to side, standing on all fours and moving her pelvis to the sound of some beautiful Indian music, and turning again and again on all four, shaking her pelvis, vomiting without inhibitions, curling into a ball, smiling a little smile; and all this without even a whimper or a complaint after more than two days without sleep, not a word about how reality was not matching up to her desired script.

Her husband and sister were great, and I myself would like to have such great support during birth. They never stopped encouraging her, not even for a moment, whispering empowering phrases to her, being quiet when she needed to rest, giving her some water or a handkerchief or whatever she needed: a hug, a pat, a massage, anything.

In the midst of all this, a third woman came storming in. This was her third birth, she had a dilation of 8 centimeters and her previous birth had been a Caesarean section. This time, her baby had been in a breech position until a week ago, when it turned around after having an acupuncture treatment. She came with her husband, who was also unusually supportive, and her doula, who had performed the acupuncture. Michal made sure via ultrasound that the baby was indeed in the correct position and then we all ran, literally, straight to the delivery room. The woman wanted to have the Dutch chair, which is a kind of stool that allows women to give birth squatting when they are otherwise unable to squat without support. Michal sat on the floor at her feet and I lay on the floor behind her so I could see properly. I felt a bit like in a garage, when you crawl under the car.

And then this woman started howling and roaring. And *aww*! This Amazon had such power. Each one of her roars could have brought down the walls of Jericho. Each time she pushed, she raised her arms like Moses in that famous battle[22] and roared loudly. Then, from beneath the chair, we saw the baby's head emerging. And when the head was out and the shoulders followed, Michal took the woman's hand and guided her to take the baby herself and lift him onto her lap. And so she did. After that, she got up, went to bed, and put the baby to her breast, but he still wanted to scream a little before he started sucking. It was a beautiful sight. The woman was lying naked on the bed, with a nice big baby in her arms; like some Greek goddess.

By the way, the baby weighed 9 lb, 4 oz. How lucky was it that she arrived at night. If she had come during the day, they would have tried to convince her to have a Caesarean section, since she had already had one in the past.

In the meantime, we struck up a conversation with the doula on pressure points, acupuncture, herbal extracts and more; a vast world of knowledge about birth, which we were given a hint of. It turns out that there are methods to relieve pain and increase contractions, and even ways to make a breeched baby turn. And while we talked, the doula went into the room where Yael was lying and started to massage her feet and hands, and taught her sister and husband how to proceed from there. Yael relaxed and gave in to the massage, and after an hour she was already 8 centimeters dilated.

It was five in the morning, and back in the nurses' station, Olivia began to teach us an African dance, the kind that moves the whole body. The movement starts at the calves, then moves to the thighs, then the hips, and then the hands join in and finally the breasts. This is a fun dance and we couldn't stop laughing as we tried to emulate

22 This refers to the battle of the Israelites and the Amalek People in the book of Exodus. When Moses raised his hands, the Israelites were winning the battle, and when he put them down, they were losing.

Olivia. Katie, who was nearly sixty years old, danced with all her heart and soul, making us roll with laughter as she shook her hips with exaggerated movements while walking.

Olivia told us about a clinic for pregnant women back in Nigeria. When women come to the clinic to monitor pregnancies that have gone past term, they have their blood pressure and temperature checked, while a staff member listens to the baby's heartbeat with a wooden fetoscope (there are not enough monitors for all of them). Then, when all the tests are finished, they stand together in two rows - thirty women along with the medical team - put on loud music and tell the women, "Come on, start dancing," or the equivalent sentence in Yoruba, and they all start dancing, moving their whole body, giving in to this intoxicating rhythm. The medical team then increases the volume and they all enjoy themselves, and within half an hour the mothers all hold their bellies and run to the delivery room with contractions.

By the way, what's wrong with Middle Eastern belly dancing, or Samba, which is a bit like this African dance? I think there used to be a female dance code that was known to women all over the world and that was given various dance expressions according to the nature and rhythms of the region, but still holds the same principle. This is an interesting topic to dig into. This kind of fleeting wisdom must be saved. I fear that in five years the same clinic in Nigeria will begin to administer Pitocin inductions and be ashamed of the "primitive methods" they once used.

Olivia tells us about all this as we dance, and the doula, who turns out to be also a dance teacher, joins us. Then Yael's sister passes by, looks at us and laughs. Even the cleaning workers and maintenance workers begin their day by looking at us and smiling.

Yael was tired, but she still rocked her pelvis. The FHR continued to beat to an African rhythm and the skies outside the window were no longer black but dark blue. A new day was dawning and with it the fear that another day has passed without her giving birth. But with dawn, also comes new hope.

I check on the woman-child whom I brought from the maternity ward with severe pain at the beginning of the shift. She is more relaxed, and says that she slept well. I connect her to a monitor and she goes back to sleep.

A few minutes before the shift ends, a woman comes in to give birth to her second child. We know her, too, from when she came for a pregnancy check. I examine her and find that she is at full dilation. Katie skips and hops with her to the delivery room, filled with joy. This is because, even though she has been a midwife for thirty-five years or so, a shift in which she did not attend a delivery is considered incomplete in her book. While handing over everything to the morning shift staff, we hear this woman scream, and when we come to her room she is already giving birth. Katie is dancing with joy; the husband is looking for the camera that he forgot to bring. Then he remembers that he actually has a cell phone and I snap the three of them.

Wow, what a shift. Eight hours of feminine presence; so diverse, enriching, empowering, strengthening and loving. Eleven different women, each one a world unto herself, and somehow, during this night, everything was woven together into a colorful quilt or a chain of shiny colored beads.

It's true; I did not receive any birth tonight. We actually laughed about it a lot - my two instructors were on duty with me and "snatched" my births from me, but I received this night as a gift tied with colorful ribbons; a precious gift indeed.

Women make plans while God watches and laughs

Many women are afraid to go to the delivery room, afraid of what might be done to them, afraid of violations of their privacy, afraid that the medical staff will not share details of their treatment with them, and most of all afraid of the unknown. In our world, we are used to planning everything, knowing everything, or at least knowing what to expect, and birth is such a different kind of process from anything else we've experienced so far. No one knows how long it will take, how it starts or how it will end.

So women sit and write a birth plan. They write what they want and how they want it to happen, and often they write with great precision exactly how they want it to happen. But the phrase "birth plan" is an oxymoron. How can you possibly plan for something that cannot be planned?

The first time I came across a birth plan it went a little like this: I went into the delivery room and reviewed the medical chart to which the birth plan was attached. It said that the woman wants to be in a delivery room with dim lights, that soft music would play in the background and that we would encourage her to change position and give her massages. I walked over and noticed that the room was lit with florescent light, while the window stood with open shutters. I asked the woman if she wanted me to darken the room and she shouted, "No, I want light!" I asked her if she wanted to change positions, listen to some music or get a massage, but she refused my suggestions and only wanted me not to touch her or rotate her. None of what she imagined seemed right when the moment of truth arrived. And this is not the only time I have encountered this; it is almost always like that. Even a woman who has already given birth a few times cannot really know how she will feel during her next birth, how she might want to be touched or even who she will want to be there with her. Reality may surprise her.

Birth plans that are styled like user manuals for the medical staff always make me squirm: *"Do not offer me any analgesics but if you do, only offer me an epidural. If a Caesarean section must be performed then insert the urine catheter after the anesthetic, unless it is a general anesthetic and in that case insert the catheter before the anesthetic."* and my favorite: *"Do not make an incision, but if you must then please stitch me using small singular stitches and not a continuous stitch."*

Whenever I read a line like this in a birth plan, which, by the way, from its prescribed format I can tell has clearly not been written by the woman but rather pulled off the Internet, I always ask the woman what she meant exactly and enjoy seeing how they blush and admit they have no idea. Yes, I admit, I too have a wicked side in me...

And the more detailed the birth plan is, the more likely it is we will end up with a Caesarean section, but not before we go through all the stations along the way: birth induction, epidurals and all kinds of other medical delicacies. I don't know why this happens, but I do have a few ideas. Maybe women who write a birth plan are people who have difficulty with not being in control and this difficulty stops and delays their delivery, and then the need for external intervention arises. Maybe the medical team gets upset because of these birth plans and decides to show the woman what they are capable of - unconsciously of course, we are also humans after all. Or maybe it just seems to me that way and I simply remember more clearly the women who had a birth plan that went wrong?

I do not know what the true reason is, but I know I've seen it happen too many times, so it is clear to me that if I give birth in a hospital I will not write a birth plan. I think that the right way to think of a future birth, as with all future events, is in terms of their basic ingredients and not in predetermined scenarios. For example, I might think about how I want to have the best support I can get, rather than name specific people who just might not be able to get to me on time, or whom at the last minute I might feel do not fit. I've seen a few birth plans that said, "I will be accompanied at birth by Sara, my best friend, and my husband Jonathan," but on the day her sister Sima was there, and Jonathan went home to rest for a while.

So to think in terms of basic ingredients is better, because when you think in full scenarios it never comes out exactly the same. Let's say I pictured a blond midwife with a braid standing to my right and I got a brunette midwife with a ponytail standing to my left. The brunette is lovely but she did not appear in my fantasies and so I am disappointed. Ingredients such as support, getting an explanation before an operation and regarding final decisions, letting go, a cozy atmosphere that suits the moment, all can be much more successful.

And besides thinking about these components, one should of course collect information. There is nothing better than knowledge to help one make the right decision and to tune one's instincts to do the right thing. Maybe in a real natural birth there is no need of knowledge - I mean a birth in the middle of the jungle, for instance - but today, when one has to deal with such a complex medical system, one must have knowledge, knowledge and more knowledge.

Ignorance is (sometimes) bliss

On the topic of ignorance in the health system, I have to let off some steam. The hospital where I work as a nurse, which is not the same hospital in which I intern as a midwife, has a really ignorant doctor who thinks she knows everything. Today I accompanied her on her ward rounds, and with every patient I got even more fired up. She gives every woman she meets absolutely horrible advice, and I have no idea where she gets it from, however it seems that she draws her knowledge from the articles in some women's magazine. For example, "To treat hemorrhoids you need to sit in a warm bath," or "Don't hold the baby too long or he'll get used to it," or "Let him feed for five minutes from each breast and that should be enough."

Moreover, she doesn't know medication dosages and asks me about every drug before she writes a prescription for the woman in question. With two drugs she did not ask for my opinion and both times she was wrong about the dosage. Now maternity wards don't actually have that many drugs to remember; all in all there is a pill for iron, several types of antibiotics and some medication for hypertension. She is disoriented, doesn't know the name of a single patient and I have to remind her which tests to administer and why. She also prescribes unnecessary treatments. For example, today I had to put a catheter in a woman simply because the doctor wanted to test the level of protein in her urine after birth, unnecessarily I might add. She immediately gives Paracetamol to every woman with a fever of 99.5°F, and in general, she is terribly messy.

That's it, I feel a little better now. But believe me; I was so furious today at having to take orders from that doctor that I almost cried from anger and resigned on the spot (honestly).

The thing is that this is not so uncommon in the medical field. I do not know why she gets on my nerves so much, since there are actually quite a few doctors like that. And what is even more frustrating is that the women patients believe and listen to her, because she is a respected doctor, and I am not, because I'm just a little nurse who does not know anything.

That's it, now I really have aired everything. So I sometimes get angry, or upset; and sometimes I even curse - oh my, I cursed in my heart so badly today; some of the curses were even vulgar. But that's okay. No need to worry about me. I have been a part of this system for several years now and am gradually learning to live with it. The people we need to worry about are you and me, when we get sick.

And when I think about it, doesn't exactly the same thing happen to all of us when we meet a dentist, mechanic, handyman, computer guy or any other person who allegedly has an area of expertise we fail to understand? How many of the people whose services we use really understand the field in which they are working? Unfortunately I have a feeling that this number is very low.

Eitan always says that this is why he loves his job - he is a violinist and a music teacher - because as a violinist, it is impossible for him to bluff. Either you can play or you cannot, and everyone can hear how good you are.

By the way, just to balance things out, there are also many doctors who are really professional, generous and good. This week, during my internship, I heard doctors say a few sentences that will forever be etched in my mind. For example, the head of the delivery room said to a woman, "I think it is best that we wait patiently for a natural birth to start on its own; what do you need an induction for?" and "Why don't you try and give birth naturally, instead of going straight to Caesarean?" and "I've learned it's best to interfere as little as possible." Apparently the Second Coming is nigh.

Oh how beautiful and special the nights are!

I had another night shift in the delivery room, and what a night it was, just wonderful. At the beginning of the shift, there were seven women in the delivery room, all after giving birth or still waiting to start labor. The evening shift midwives greeted me and apologized, "We've already dealt with all the births for you." "Never mind," I consoled myself, "soon a lot of women will come to give birth."

During the first hour, we dealt with transfers: transferring women to the maternity ward after giving birth; transferring some patients to the emergency room and others to be discharged from the front desk. When I was at the front desk, two women turned up, almost simultaneously, after having their waters break. Both had no dilation or contractions and we thought, well, let's admit them to the ward and tomorrow morning we'll see what to do with them. But this night had other plans for them.

While we were admitting the first woman, her contractions started. They were mild at first and not really noticeable, but pretty soon they got stronger. We gave her a quick check with the monitor and she went to walk around a bit and have a bath. The second woman we transferred to the maternity ward anyway, just for her to come back half an hour later with strong contractions and 4 centimeters dilation.

The two women, who were not aware of each other at all, progressed at the same pace and very rapidly. At first I was with both of them, but at a certain moment one of the women didn't want me to leave the room because she felt the need to push and it seemed that she would give birth soon. I stayed with her and another midwife went to be with the other woman.

What a beautiful birth she had! She stood beside the bed and hugged her husband during each contraction while shaking her pelvis. It all happened so quickly. As soon as I finished preparing everything, she said she already felt the need to push. I examined her and she was 9 centimeters dilated. I suggested she might want to stand on all fours so she would feel less pressure until she is fully dilated. She then stood on all fours and hugged her husband who was standing next to the bed with each contraction. She even hugged me once. This is a little strange – you've just met a woman and after an hour you're hugging her tight, her face in your hair. Strange, and yet also somehow completely natural.

Within a few minutes, she was already fully dilated, but then she was suddenly struck by some terrible fear and everything stopped. Michal, my instructor, said to her softly, "you are holding yourself back, you need to let go." And after she relaxed, within two contractions she gave birth. During her contractions, she got really wild in bed – it looked like a kind of storm of legs, arms and sheets. Through the whole ordeal, I was trying to "protect the perineum," as midwives say (which means to try and prevent a rapid descent of the head in order to avoid tears), without having much success, but with a lot of joy. From within this storm came a charming and calm baby who was greeted with tears of happiness, and a minute or two after she gave birth we heard the cries of the baby born to the other woman in the room next door.

I was so glad that this is how it ended, because sometimes when the waters break and there are no contractions, we encounter problems that require inductions and antibiotics. It was also very heartwarming to see that these two women arrived and gave birth at the very same time. It was as if their babies had arranged to meet each other.

And so my shift went by, and the sky began to lighten up a bit on the horizon, and another mother-to-be arrived. She was an ultra-Orthodox woman, even ultra-ultra-Orthodox if there is such a thing. She lives in one of the surrounding towns known for its ultra-Orthodox Jewish community, a joyful and conservative community where women start to give birth at the age of fifteen and it's not uncommon to see a twenty-year-old woman having her third child.

Anyway, this woman wanted a natural birth and did not want much of anything the hospital had to offer. Do you know what a hospitalization form looks like? It says, "I agree to be admitted to this hospital and agree to the following: fetal monitoring, induction, the administering of an IV drip, and so on." There is a possibility to mark what you do and do not want, and this woman had marked that she wanted... nothing.

She asked for a corner room next to the shower (not that she would have a chance to use it, as things turned out) and in the meantime, she put on the clothes she had prepared in advance for her birth: a full outfit that included shoes, socks, a long skirt, long-sleeved shirt buttoned all the way to the top and a head covering. She stood in her room, next to the bed, and during contractions she took deep breaths and held her hip.

I asked her if she had any special requests regarding her delivery, and she said she wanted to try and give birth using a birth chair. I went out and cheerfully brought back the chair. She obviously did not want any tests to be done on her and so I told her that if she felt any pressure she should immediately call me back to the room. In the meantime, I ran and ate a peach yogurt (that's all a hospital kitchen has in the middle of the night) and then her husband came to tell me that she was feeling pressure. I gave up the peach yogurt and ran back to her. She was fully dilated.

I put a cushion under the seat of her chair; she sat on it, still with all her clothes, socks and everything, while I sat down on a stool beside her. She agreed that we could hear a little heartbeat on the monitor, just for half a second, and right after, without waiting, the baby's head was already showing.

When you attend a birth in a birthing chair you actually "attend" it, because you really don't have to do anything. Even if you want to "protect the perineum" there is nothing you can do. So I was just waiting with open arms for the baby so that when it emerged it would not fall on its head. When it came down, I grabbed the baby immediately and placed it in its mother's arms.

I forgot to say that this woman has four sons at home and that she did not know the gender of the fetus. So as soon as the baby was born, we saw that it was actually a baby girl and the room was filled with cheers of joy - from all the midwives who had gathered to see a birth on a birthing chair, from the mother and from the father, who had waited behind a curtain.

Then she got up from the chair with the umbilical cord still attached and the baby in her arms, and went to the bed. The placenta came out and she started to breastfeed the baby instead of taking medications to contract the uterus. It was just a beautiful birth. Ah! I almost forgot to write that the amniotic sac did not burst until the head was out and I actually saw it burst and it was just beautiful.

So this was a night of women who had fast and easy deliveries; a night of women whose bodies knew how to give birth and who themselves believed in this knowledge and this wonderful ability... a calm and starry night.

Wait a moment, all this happened yesterday and I didn't even tell you what happened today

I'm a little hesitant, because while every day in the delivery room is special and every birth is an experience unto itself, the details might sound a bit repetitive, or maybe even... boring?

I hope I'm not boring you, but I really feel like I want to tell about each and every birth; what the mother looked like, at what rate the birth progressed, what her husband said, what kind of look she had in her eyes, how she dealt with the pain, if it was hard for her and how she overcame this, how she jumped from 6 centimeters dilation to full dilation – or how her birth stopped progressing suddenly, how she was laughing…or crying, and how the baby was born and how much he weighed, what he looked like, how much he cried, and so on and so on. Thousands of details that I feel are stored in me and which I want to tell. So what should I do with all these stories?

Today, for example, I attended three births, which were so different from one another and yet all so beautiful and good.

With the first birth, I had met the mother-to-be at the beginning of my shift, after she was already in full dilation and had received an epidural shot. She was twenty-one and giving birth for the first time. She was really sweet and joyful. Her husband was also very happy and both of them were really excited about becoming parents. Despite the epidural and despite the fact that she did not feel anything -- seriously, not a thing -- she did just great and progressed rapidly. And soon she gave birth to a beautiful and sweet baby girl. Oh, how happy they were to see her! And this young mother, young enough that even I could be her mother, had this lightheaded joyfulness that very young women sometimes have, without the heavy-handed concerns that come with age.

The second birth started with a thick meconial water break. This was the woman's third birth and it progressed very slowly. The woman was in a lot of pain but could not be given an epidural because she was not dilated enough. Later on, the monitor showed heart rate deceleration and a look of concern crept onto the doctors' faces, because her dilation was still only 5 centimeters and, like I said, she was progressing very slowly. But then, within ten minutes, she reached full dilation and after three contractions, the baby was born, covered with a thick layer of vernix and not caring one bit that his amniotic fluid was thick meconial. Amazingly, the pediatrician did not care much about it either, and the newborn stayed with his mom to breastfeed.[23]

The third birth was completely different. It was the woman's second birth. She progressed quickly and reached a dilation of 8

---

23 A few words about Meconium liquor: In most cases, the infant passes stool for the first time in the first day after birth. This stool is called meconium and is not the result of the baby's breastfeeding but the intestinal secretions during pregnancy. Sometimes the baby excretes the meconium while in the womb. This can be due to some sort of distress he experiences, sometimes even a slight and meaningless distress - for example, a momentary pressure on the umbilical cord. The rate of appearance of meconium liquor increases in post-term pregnancies, meaning pregnancies that go on after week forty-one of the pregnancy. When the water breaks, we see that the color is not transparent-white but yellow, green or brown. As the baby spends more time in the womb after meconium secretion, the more likely it is he will inhale it into his lungs and therefore it is recommended that induction be carried out immediately following the passing of meconium liquor (when the water is clean, it is possible to wait a few days for the birth to develop naturally). Immediately after the birth, the pediatrician will decide, according to the newborn's state, whether it is necessary to perform a suction of the airways or not. A very small percentage of babies will develop, within a few hours, a condition called 'meconium aspiration syndrome,' which is characterized by difficulty of breathing to varying degrees and which in rare cases can endanger the baby's life.

centimeters and then got stuck in that state for nearly three hours. The baby was in an occipital posterior position (which means he was facing up instead of down) which was perhaps the reason for the lack of progress in labor. I tried to convince the woman to come down from the bed and walk around a little so the baby could turn around and come down, but she refused and only wanted an epidural. The doctor finally agreed to her request and called an anesthesiologist.

The woman got off the bed in order to move into a different room where it would be more convenient to perform the epidural anesthesia. In the new room, she was lying on the bed and we connected her to the monitor. I went to get a bag of IV fluids and when I came back her husband had just left the room. He was nervous and looking for me with a sense of urgency. "I don't know what's going on, but I think maybe she's about to give birth!" he said. I entered the room and saw half a head crowning out. I quickly put on gloves and got there just in time to give the baby to his mother, because the rest of the work she did all by herself.

It was amazing to see how the moment of giving birth erased all the pain she had felt up to this point. Her face was beaming great happiness and she immediately started breastfeeding her little baby boy (who weighed 5 lb, 8 oz).

This is a summary of the day's events. But, you see, that's not the whole story. What about the expressions on the faces of the women, the sounds they made, how they moved, how their bellies looked, what shape the umbilical cord was...? There are a huge number of details that, probably because of the intensity of the experience, become etched in my mind and repeat themselves like a movie playing over and over. After a couple of days, some images remain bright and lucid, while others get mixed up in that great pot of my birth experiences.

And another small thing: the moment I love most is the one just before birth. There are a few adults in the room: the mother, the midwife and possibly another man or woman; a break between contractions; stillness. At that moment, I always try to imagine the room as it will be in a few minutes, when a new person will have joined us; tiny, screaming, bluish pink, kicking his legs and hands. Everything is going to change radically; the atmosphere, sounds, feelings, smells... everything. And the world is going to change a little too, since suddenly it will contain a new person who wasn't there before. And the moment before that, that quiet moment, always reminds me of the wonderful world that God created.

So... if it doesn't bore you, I have to tell you about another birth that happened yesterday

We arrived for the evening shift and a woman just walked in, about to give birth for the second time, with 3 centimeters dilation. We gave her a quick reading with the monitor and suggested she walk around a bit. At first she wasn't keen on doing so, but within a minute or two she stood up and walked down the hall. We suggested that she also bounce a bit on the physiotherapy ball, but her husband put his foot down and said: "No ball!" I have no idea why.

In the meantime, I went to check on another woman and after about twenty minutes, I came back. She coped amazingly well with her contractions. During each contraction, she stayed quite composed and it could hardly be seen on the outside that she has any pain at all; nothing more than a small shake of her pelvis.

After a few minutes, I went into her room and found her on the bed. Just as I entered, she made kind of an "Ahhh..." sound. I helped her quickly take her panties off and not a minute later, the amniotic sac appeared, intact and completely out of her vagina. I was so excited! It had been my dream to see such a birth, where the water didn't break until after the baby had arrived.

My instructor also heard the "Ahhh..." and was in the room with me half a minute later. Then that quiet and composed woman suddenly became a raging tigress. Within three to four contractions, she gave birth to a cute little baby girl, and it took her less than an hour from the time she reached the delivery room.

Later that evening, I attended the Caesarean of a woman whose birth did not progress fast enough and she constantly asked for surgery. I really do not understand why women think that surgery is so much fun. In my work in the maternity ward, I see how tormented women are after a Caesarean, how they can barely get out of the bed and how they find it hard to even hold the baby and breastfeed.

Finally, it was decided to have surgery after all and I went into the operating theater to receive the baby. A midwife doesn't have a very important role in an operating theater, only to help in all sorts of little things, like fastening the doctor's sterile gown, directing the light or inserting a urinary catheter. The main thing is to take the baby from the surgeon and to take care of it from that moment onward. Usually it is not the most exciting thing in the world, but this time it was. The operation was carried out under general anesthetic because the woman had a back problem that prevented the administering of a local anesthetic. A few moments before the anesthetic kicked in, I asked her if there was anything special that she wanted done with the baby. She was a bit surprised by the question. She thought a little and finally requested that we greet it by saying "Welcome." After the anesthesia did its trick, I passed that request on to the surgical team and for some reason expected to hear them laugh at me or make some cynical remark about it, but instead they took the request very seriously and when the baby was born, he received a wholehearted "welcome" from the entire staff -- two nurses, three doctors and me. The goodwill of people is everywhere to be found.

Meanwhile, a woman who was giving birth for the fourth time arrived with full dilation. She gave birth on the birth chair and unfortunately I was not present at her birth. After the birth, Michal, my instructor, who delivered her, followed the woman into the bathroom. When I went to give them a towel, I opened the bathroom door just a crack and what I saw was just heartwarming: the woman was sitting on a step in the tub, and Michal was pouring warm water on her back. The bathroom light was low, but their faces were lit from the inside as they chatted quietly and happily - such a lovely sight. They looked like a mother and daughter or two sisters or longtime friends. I have no doubt there was another presence in the room, that of love.

I put the towel on a chair and quietly shut the door. I felt full of joy.

I finally understand what it means to be a real apprentice

This understanding came during a birth I attended this week. It was a really nice birth and I was there with Katie, one of my instructors. When we arrived for the morning shift, we were told that there was a wonderful woman waiting for us. During her last checkup she had been 6 centimeters dilated and she was giving birth for the second time. At that time, she was the only woman in the delivery room, so we were able to be with her all the time.

We entered the room and each introduced ourselves. The woman was kind of a Greek goddess: over six feet tall, with olive skin, and very robust. She told us she worked as a lifeguard at a pool. Her man was hugging her from behind and rubbing her back. She walked around the room restlessly due to her contractions and immediately shared with us her worries over whether or not to have an epidural. During her first birth, she had had an epidural, and she wanted to try without this time, even though she was not sure if she would be able to handle it. She had just had a nice, long shower and the monitor showed that everything was in order. We said, let's examine you and then you'll decide. I checked her and she had a dilation of 8 centimeters. The husband didn't trust my ruling and asked that Katie check as well. She checked and approved it: 8 centimeters.

"But how much longer will it take?!" the woman asked. As I have already said, this is the million-dollar question. So I begin to answer, "Well… you cannot really know exactly...". But Katie stopped me, and said it seemed she would give birth within half an hour - a forecast that half an hour later would turn out to be amazingly accurate. She decided to try without an epidural.

So this Amazon sat on a huge physiotherapy ball (the biggest I've seen so far) they had brought from home, and the next twenty minutes passed with all of us making grunts and growls and other low noises, and with each contraction we all competed over who could make the lowest sound. It was so nice to hear how she started at a certain pitch, with the tone of her voice becoming lower and lower as the contraction progressed, until it didn't sound at all like a human voice but like an ancient Aboriginal growl.

Imagine this weird scenario: a contraction starts, the woman makes noises and moves, I'm sitting on a stool next to her and growl at her, Katie stands over her and hugs her, or rather, the woman grabs hold of her, while Katie tries to hold back and the man stands behind her, rubbing and growling as well.

In between contractions the woman kept asking, "So how long do I have? What will I do if it goes on for hours like this? I can't take it... and how will I know how to push and when? When I had an epidural, I felt nothing... how many more contractions do I have?" and so on. But every time, another contraction stopped us and there wasn't a lot of time to discuss these questions. We could only tell her that she would know when it was time to push. But she did not believe us and repeatedly asked how she would know.

"What position do you want to give birth in?" I asked. She didn't really know. The man suggested she do it standing up, Katie suggested she do it on the ball and I suggested the Dutch chair. She had never heard of that, so I brought it and we decided that just before birth she would choose what to do, according to what seemed the most convenient at the moment.

In this way another five minutes passed, when suddenly she jumped up from the ball, with amniotic fluid gushing out, and cried: "I need to go to the toilet!" We all cheered her, laughing and said, "It's time."

For the special occasion she chose the Dutch chair, sat on it and started pushing. Katie sat next to her, her man behind her and

I underneath. Meanwhile two other midwives entered: the Dutch birth chair is still considered some sort of innovation in this delivery room and all midwives are interested in how it works exactly.

She did not want me to examine her, and I did not think it was really necessary, so I didn't. Then she said, "But I'm fully dilated, right?" I told her that it looked as if she was but if she wanted I could check. "You're just confusing me with all these options!" She said and she was right, so I just checked her, and the baby's head was "right here," as midwives say.

During the next contraction a string of membranes came out, and with the contraction that followed came the head and then the body, and hop – the baby went straight to its Mama's hands. It was quick and beautiful: the woman sat on a low chair, with the baby wrapped in membrane in her hands and the man's arms wrapped around her from behind. Both touched the baby and kissed him. It seemed as if the whole room faded around them.

After a few minutes, she got up with the baby and went to bed, where the placenta came out intact. Only then did I cut the umbilical cord. In a very strange way, this birth hadn't even involved a drop of blood, except for what emerged wrapped and packaged in the placenta.

We left the baby in his mother's arms for an hour and a half, and only then did we take him to be weighed. There was a tiny tear that didn't need sewing and after two and a half hours, she went to take a shower while her sweet baby, who just sucked and sucked and sucked, was brought to the nursery for just a brief moment. She got out of the shower and went to the maternity ward in a wheelchair under her own power... she was just amazing.[24]

---

24 A few words about breastfeeding in the delivery room. Most healthy babies will be interested in breastfeeding within a quarter to half an hour after birth. The breastfeeding reflex during that time is most powerful and there

I thought that this was the way it should be. A woman gives birth by herself and does not lose energy in the process. On the contrary, the process strengthens and invigorates her.

Two other small things: the first is about the man, who was supportive and loving in an extraordinary way, but after birth became a bit suspicious and fundamentally opposed to everything I proposed. When I suggested that his wife take a shower, for example, he firmly said "No!" and it wasn't so pleasant, especially after this beautiful birth experience. His wife however replied, "Actually, I'd be glad to." But I think this came from being overprotective, rather than genuine suspicion. I felt it was a little hard for him that I was an intern and not a midwife, and mostly because I was with Katie, who is an amazing midwife who has delivered babies for more years than I've been alive.

And this leads me to the second thing: this actually was the first birth where I really felt I was an apprentice, in the sense of trying to catch the spark that someone else has. I felt like I just drank in every little nuance from Katie, every word, every look, every touch, every laugh and every encouragement, every change in tone and every decision. I kept repeating to myself, "Watch her and do exactly as she does." Wow, what an artist she is!

So if I look at it from the perspective of this man, I too would want my wife to be delivered by Katie and not some intern; and when I realized this, I felt that his responses weren't so hard on me.

---

is a greater chance of success in breastfeeding. There are many benefits for breastfeeding in the delivery room for the mother and the baby. Breastfeeding causes the secretion of oxytocin in the mother's body, which helps contraction of the uterus and prevents excessive bleeding after birth. For the infant, breastfeeding prevents a drop in blood sugar, helps calm him down, increases his sense of security, helps warm him (since a mother's breasts are warmer than the rest of her body), reinforces the bonding process between the mother and her baby and increases the chances of successful breastfeeding in the future.

At the end he told me, "There are some amazing midwives here. If you learn from them, you too will be a wonderful midwife." This is definitely a sentence that might annoy some, but I agreed with it with all my heart.

Apparently it is just like chicken...

I mean the perineum. We showed up at school for a stitching workshop that was a combination of Martha Stewart and the Adams Family.

Maybe I should explain a bit. Nowadays in Israel, midwives, at least in hospitals, do not perform stitching, but not long ago there was an initiative for them to replace doctors in doing that task. Why? Because it is much more logical for the midwife, who accompanies the mother-to-be, takes care of her for hours, attends the birth and sometimes performs an incision, to also be able to stitch what has been cut or torn. A full treatment from A to Z, and not as is the case today, when suddenly a doctor emerges, someone who may not have met the woman before, and the mother has to wait with her feet up as the doctor immediately settles down in between her legs...

Besides, why shouldn't midwives give stitches anyway? It only increases their skills, and as a result, increases their autonomy, allowing them, for example, to stitch tears during home births, instead of referring the woman to a hospital for that. In countries where midwives also give stitches, everyone is more satisfied: the women, midwives and doctors. Just between us - doctors hate to give stitches. They drop this task on the interns, who have enough work on their shoulders as it is.

So in short, it started some time ago. They gave this workshop to midwives in one of the largest hospitals in Tel Aviv, and put them to work. It was very successful, but just before the program expanded to other places, the doctors' union got cold feet and froze the whole process. The absurdity is that those who opposed it were the specialists, the ones who do the least amount of stitching. By the way, in the hospital where they gave the workshop, midwives still stitch. Despite all this, the intention is probably for us to perform this procedure sometime in the future, so we'd better be prepared for it.

The workshop included a lecture from a doctor about when, how and why we give stitches; when we cannot give stitches and have to call a doctor, and when we can, which is in most cases. After the lecture, we got some string and practiced making knots. It's not terribly complicated, but not entirely simple either. You need to learn how to tie a regular and reverse knot with one hand. The reason for making the knot with one hand is that when you make a stitch in the vagina there isn't room for both hands.

After about two hundred knots, we moved on to knotting with a "needle holder," a kind of small plier with which you push the needle into the tissue. It is much easier and feels "professional." Then we moved on to sponges. We each received a sponge, gave it an episiotomy and then stitched it up. What fun, we did not hurt it at all and the sponge did not move or shout as we stitched.

Finally, the funny/disgusting stage came. Each one of us brought a whole grocery store chicken from home, a cutting board and a scissors. We gave our birds vaginas and rectum-shaped holes, and then gave them episiotomies. The chickens got treated for severe bleeding and we practiced everything we had learned in theory. It was a rather bizarre situation. Imagine thirty students sitting around tables, each with a chicken on the table in front of her, as she cuts and repairs it, showing off her neat little stitches (mine by the way were very nice. You think I'm bragging?) Occasionally, someone stitched a flap onto the chicken's breast to try something. The funniest thing was when we gave the chicken a rectal exam to see that we didn't accidentally sew its rectum.

At the end of the day, there were thirty ragged birds, full of scars that will never heal despite their perfect stitching. I took some birds home; one of them provided entertainment for our dog, while another fell into the hands of a friend, who said he did not see any reason not to eat it ... ugh.

I left the training thoroughly repulsed at any form of chicken, and could only wish that the doctor had had us train on bread or chocolate. Maybe it would have put me off them once and for all.

By the way, the course was attended by a good number of home birth midwives, who came to learn how to stitch or to improve their technique. It was such fun to listen to their conversations, to envy them and admire them secretly at heart. I was captivated by every movement they made.

So now we know how to stitch, or at least how to stitch chickens. I'm not so sure about a vagina or a perineum. I hope to have the opportunity to practice; otherwise this skill will be forgotten.

By the way, did you know that doctors don't do this workshop before they start to give stitches? At best there is someone who helps them test the water a little. They do not train on sponges or poultry, they train on women.

Two nights straight in the delivery room

And the two were so different from one another - as if they existed in two different realities. This diversity is part of what is so delightful about the delivery room, although the first night of the two I would have passed up.

On the first night, we arrived for our shift, which was destined to be the longest shift of the year, due to a switch from daylight savings during the night. Although on many occasions midwives stay a few more hours to attend the delivery of a woman whom they had attended to during the previous shift, when the process is forced, it suddenly seems very long and tiring. In the delivery room, there were two women, one with full dilation and a second with 4 centimeters; both giving birth for the first time.

I immediately joined the woman who was at full dilation. She had been at full dilation for seventy-five minutes, pushing and screaming, but nothing progressed. She pushed just the way she should, but the head wasn't pressed and was still high in the canal. If you'd have asked me, we could have let her continue at full dilation for another hour or two, or three, until the head descended, but unfortunately this is not how it works...

First, she herself constantly said, "Get him out of me! I can't take it anymore! I'm going to die! I can't take it anymore! Get him out of me! Give me surgery! I can't take it anymore!" She had been given analgesics two hours ago and it was very difficult to calm her down. Second, the FHR didn't look very good and we couldn't let things go on for too long. And third, there is a protocol in the delivery room that after two hours at full dilation, the staff has to intervene. It is a protocol that exists in all delivery rooms in the country and the rationale is that the chance for any progress declines over time (although there are women who give birth after five hours in full dilation), while the risk of complications gradually increases.

She pushed for another hour without any progress. We then called the doctor and started that hectic race to prepare for a Caesarean section, just to be on the safe side. Another doctor was invited and we informed the operating theater. In the meantime, we continued to try getting her to push in a variety of ways: we took out urine with a catheter, because often this is what holds up the baby, and we helped her to change positions, but nothing moved. Suddenly, something did move a little and the head was low enough to try to vacuum. And indeed, a short and relatively mild vacuum got this cute little baby out.

After the birth, the doctor stitched her for over an hour because she had a deep tear in her vagina, which might have been caused by the vacuum but probably occurred earlier, and maybe that's what allowed the baby to descend after so many hours.

The woman, by the way, was very sweet and it looked as if she was taking it all quite easily. Perhaps the analgesics did their part? I do not know. Three hours later, I saw her breastfeeding in the ward. Anyway, midwives generally like to attend a delivery they worked hard on for several hours and don't like some physician to just come and get the baby out with a vacuum. And besides, the vacuum is such an intrusive intervention. I have not yet formed an opinion as to whether it is preferable to surgery or not. I should think about it and get more experience of it.

Well, so this birth was over, and in the meantime the other woman had progressed to 8 centimeters. She had had an epidural a few hours before and she wanted another because it had begun to wear off and it was very painful for her. We tried to convince her that this was not recommended, but she would not listen, she wanted an epidural. Well, we called the anesthesiologist who also tried to persuade her not to do it, since she was almost fully dilated, and it was actually time to stop the epidural and start pushing, but she insisted. We should have refused...

So she got another epidural and a minute later, the FHR dropped down to fifty and stayed that way. Within five minutes she found herself in an operating theater with a catheter, oxygen, and three tense doctors. In the end, the pulse recovered somewhat but still did not look good, and the head was very high, so it was decided to operate. The baby was a bit large and had a big Caput succedaneum (swelling in the scalp caused by an edema). This is usually the result of a baby who entered the birth canal at a bad angle.

So this was the day before yesterday, and the midwives were really frustrated, tired and upset. Towards dawn, we took all the women who were post-delivery back to the maternity ward and just dropped, deflated, on chairs until the morning shift woke us up.

Don't think a delivery room is filled only with nice stories, excitement and natural births. Although even with hard births there are beautiful moments, excitement, the ushering of new life into this world, and families who are happy. I guess that this is a glass half-empty/glass half-full kind of situation.

The second night was different. It was a night of women who came and gave birth; came and gave birth; came and gave birth. It started when we arrived for our shift and found that the midwife who works with my instructor and me had just finished attending a birth. "Well," I said with a smile, "it's a good thing you did, because I will attend all the others." You see, students have the right of way in those matters. In practice it turned out she had the most births in the shift.

A few minutes later, a woman who was giving birth for the fifth time, and who was renowned for her fast labor progress, turned up, and I got to attend. We quickly entered the delivery room, since she progressed from 4 centimeters to 7 within four minutes. This woman was amazing. She handled her contractions in a withdrawn way. With every contraction, she went into some inner place in herself and didn't move or make a sound. She endured the contractions just by concentrating deeply. Between contractions, she smiled and talked. She had already been through every kind of delivery in the past: twins, a baby in breech position and a big baby who weighed 9.5 pounds. In short, I call this, "a woman who knows how to give birth."

But despite all this, the birth did not progress and was stuck at 9 centimeters dilation for about an hour. In truth, an hour at that kind of dilation is entirely natural during birth, but in terms of this particular woman it was a long time.

Michal and I came to the conclusion that the baby was upside down, meaning with her face looking up instead of down, and indeed all the signs for it were there. We tried to help the baby turn around by changing the woman's position, but without much success. The woman was already at full dilation, pushing and pushing and pushing, and since she was accustomed to giving birth within fifteen minutes, it really was the longest and most difficult birth she had experienced – although it took only two and a half hours altogether.

Eventually, the baby turned around just before she came out. We actually saw it happen. It was a beautiful birth, without any interference in the end, and so we were happy -- especially after the frustrating shift we had experienced the previous night. This couple was so nice. They were quite young, and just wanted to have a lot of children because they love them so much. They showed me a picture of their four other children, sitting or standing on top of their father. Now the new baby girl will join this happy group.

As we attended this birth, another woman came in and gave birth within half an hour, and then another woman who gave birth within half an hour. These two births were attended with great joy by the other midwife.

Well, things settled down a bit, and at four in the morning we finally had time to drink some herb tea. We rested a bit until five in the morning and then came a knock on the door. We looked outside and saw two Ultra-Orthodox women, one of whom (the one with the big belly) was noticeably restless. "Well," I said, "it seems we are about to have another birth."

They came in, a mother and her daughter, who was giving birth for the second time. She had strong and frequent and we rushed her to the delivery room. But here I was faced with a little shock. The woman was only sixteen years old and she had had her first baby when she was fourteen. Just think how old she had to have been when she married... It was really hard for me to understand and accept.

Imagine yourself giving birth at the age of fourteen (in eighth grade!), and again at the age of sixteen. Imagine living with a man and sustaining a marriage from the age of thirteen. If she goes the way of her sister, then by the age of twenty-five she will already have seven children...

She was scared and wanted her mother to hug her all the time. Within three-quarters of an hour, she was already holding the baby in her arms, and all in all she did really well. She was also one of those women who just know how to give birth. It seemed to be only I, and call me judgmental if you will, who wished she had not found that out at such a young age.

So this is how this night ended, and I was so pumped with adrenaline and thoughts about girls who give birth that I wasn't even tired when I drove home, and thus didn't need to stop at some intersection to sleep for a while, as is sometimes the case. I do not think midwifery is a "beautiful" profession in the romantic sense, as many think, but it is certainly varied, interesting, challenging, frustrating, educational, maturing and just the right profession for me.

The solo

This wasn't supposed to happen, but I received a delivery all by myself, without anyone else in the room, simply because the other three midwives on the shift were also attending deliveries at exactly the same time. It was less scary than I thought, and filled me with a sense of pride: Here I go - I am a real midwife now! Maybe it's like a pilot's first solo flight. It is clear that he still has a lot to learn, but after this solo flight, everything seems different.

Today I counted how many births I've delivered so far and I got to eighty (but who's counting, right?). This is but a drop in the ocean of experience, but it's my drop and I'm happy about it. Moreover, as a student I do not have many more births to attend, because I only have five more shifts in my internship, out of which one or two will be dedicated to working in the IVF unit.

I need to start saying goodbye to the delivery room, which means saying goodbye to the smell of amniotic fluid that is always in the air, mixed with the smell of disinfectants, the smell of hormone-saturated blood, wheat germ oil and other birth aromas. The faint smell of amniotic fluid will always symbolize for me "the smell of a delivery room." This also means saying goodbye to this wonderful realm, where women reach their limits and surpass them again and again and again; where women undergo experiences that are life-changing at times; where women become mothers and goddesses.

The delivery room is also a realm of unending pain, the realm of fear, terror, fatigue, despair, joy, happiness, hope, delight. A realm where everything is exposed and nothing can be swept under the rug, not the nature of your relationship with your partner, not your fears, not your weaknesses and strengths, not the shape of your body or the fluids that come out of it; everything is exposed.

So in my heart, I start to say goodbye to all the little things. It will take a few months before they will become a part of my life again. Katie says that I am missing only two crucial things needed to conclude my training - one is experience and the other is giving birth myself.

How fast can a delivery help form a deep relationship with a stranger?

It was an evening shift, which started at three in the afternoon. We arrived for our shift and moved from room to room, when suddenly there was an unmistakable shout: someone was about to give birth. My instructor told me, "Run." So I ran.

The baby was born at fourteen minutes past three, so I had fourteen minutes to meet the woman and her husband, introduce myself, examine her, encourage her to push and receive this wet and wriggling baby; very strange. *"Hi, I'm Dana, what's your name? Do you feel the urge to push? Then push..."* Maybe this is not the exact way it played out, but that was the general idea. Within half a minute, we were closer than anyone could imagine.

After birth, women stay in the delivery room for another two hours. We had a chance then to get to know each other a little, but this was a different kind of introduction. It came from a much deeper place, as if we had been long-time friends who were now catching up, while smiling and laughing; I'm teasing her a little about the funny way she was shouting when I pressed on her belly to check her uterus, which reminded me of an opera singer. And she is rolling with laughter and asks me questions about me, which I answer, and the conversation goes on like that, even with her nice husband... and all this with a woman I do not know, despite the fact that normally I am shy and introverted, and find it difficult to open up to new people. But I might need to change my view of myself. It seems to me that, without me noticing, a lot of things have changed.

A few hours later, I was at the front desk. There were two women there: one who was about to give birth and one who wasn't. The one that wasn't asked me where the women who give birth are, so I told her that right next to her, for example, there was a woman who is about to give birth. She looked at her and said, "Really? She doesn't look like it!" but a second later, the woman had a contraction and looked very much like she was about to give birth. It was her third time giving birth and every contraction was more powerful than the last. Within five minutes, she could no longer stand still and during each contraction she just had to hug someone (me) and dance around a bit. She did not know me before either, but again, it did not matter at all. It was very pleasant to dance like that in front of her swollen belly and feel it stiffening during each contraction.

When she got a private room she wouldn't stay there alone for a moment (she's right, isn't she?) and had to lean on, hold on and move around with each contraction. I was with her in the room for three hours, until she gave birth. She did not want anything for the pain and her endorphins[25] levels were crazily high. She was so dazed that whoever entered the room said, "Oh, I see she got sedatives..." When her dilation was at 4 centimeters, she was still able to talk on the phone about family matters, such as her children, laundry, cooking, transportation, chores and so on. But as her labor progressed, there was a radical change. Between contractions she slept or talked nonsense and during contractions she was in pain,

---

25 Endorphins - When a woman experiences pain in childbirth, the body produces endorphins, which are natural substances that relieve pain. As the pain increases, so does the secretion of endorphins. This is why women who do not take painkillers will often be really drowsy between contractions and will later tell of a different sense of awareness during labor.

but in a distant way, as if in her own world. Every time I let go of her hand to leave, she opened her eyes wide and said in Arabic, "But come back soon." And again I was amazed at how quickly such a deep connection and dedication, which cannot be found anywhere else, can form.

The midwife's nightmare

Maybe my dream of becoming a big fat midwife with white hair tied in a bun will come true faster than I imagined - at least regarding the white hair.

Tonight I attended a delivery that ended with shoulder dystocia. This is a situation where the shoulders get stuck after the head is already born; or in other words, the head is outside, the body is stuck inside. This is a very scary and stressful situation; one of those emergency situations no midwife wants to have, but they still happen.

This lovely couple arrived shortly after the start of my shift. The woman was giving birth for the second time, with 5 centimeters dilation and painful contractions. Weight assessment suggested a big baby, about eight and a half pounds. During her first birth, she had delivered a six and a half pound baby. Well, okay; overall, this is not a very unusual weight. So you file this fact in your head and continue. The delivery progressed quickly, and at 8 centimeters dilation, the woman really wanted an epidural. The anesthesiologist just happened to be in the next room treating another woman, so soon after, the woman was given an epidural and the birth continued. Her waters broke by themselves, the head descended and everything was great.

At some point she was already fully dilated and felt pressure and the need to push. The head came down pretty fast and we were happy because we remembered that we were dealing with a big baby here, and a lot of times in such births if the head doesn't descend and the birth gets stuck, it's a sign that later there might be shoulder dystocia. Within two or three contractions, the head was already crowning and the woman pushed, and pushed, and pushed, and pushed and pushed. And with every passing moment, more and more and more of the head appeared; a huge head that just did not end.

At this point, Michal called another midwife and doctor to our aid. We had not yet encountered shoulder dystocia, but we feared we were about to have one. The first rule of shoulder dystocia: quickly call for help. I knew this because I was going to have a test about it in three days.

Finally, this huge head came out, suggesting a huge body would follow, well over our previous estimations. But the body was slow to come out. The three of us jumped on her (the McRoberts maneuver and Supra pubic pressure) and Whoops! Out came the shoulders.[26]

The baby was born not in the best of conditions. She was blue, flaccid, not crying and barely breathing. We immediately cut the umbilical cord and the baby was handed over to a pediatrician, who had been called in advance. Meanwhile, in the delivery room, the

---

26 A few words about shoulder dystocia: There are all sorts of maneuvers designed to help dislodge a stuck baby. The first thing you try is the McRoberts maneuver, which means that you raise both of the woman's legs at the same time. This position extends the pelvic aperture and helps the pubic bone, under which the upper shoulder is trapped, to move and release the stuck shoulder. In 90% of cases it is sufficient. Supra Pubic Pressure is the exertion of pressure over the woman's pubis (the pubic bone, which is one of the pelvic bones). What you are actually doing is pressing on the baby's shoulder and trying to push it under the pubis. It is important to press from the right direction, which is from the baby's back. Then there are all sorts of maneuvers that include bilateral episiotomy (argh!); reaching in with your hand and turning the baby or pulling one of his hands; the Gaskin maneuver (named after Ina May Gaskin, the famous midwife), which involves the woman standing on all fours; through to the Zavanelli maneuver, which is to push the baby back in and rush the woman to surgery (sounds surreal and is rarely used). There are even more brutal ways. I do not have to specify them... right? Shoulder dystocia is not called "the midwife's nightmare" for nothing.

drama continued. The husband turned pale and almost fainted. We had to elevate his feet and wake him up. As this was going on the woman was shouting, "Why doesn't she cry? Why doesn't she cry?" and I wondered myself why the hell didn't she cry!

This went on for a very short time in total, but you know how those moments are; it seems that every minute is an eternity. After a few minutes, the baby recovered and was placed in the arms of her mother, who was so happy. The father recovered and took the traditional post-birth pictures. After the placenta was delivered, I was afraid I had something akin to a fourth-degree tear on my hands. Yet soon it became clear that the woman had not a scratch on her and there was no need for stitches, even though the baby ultimately weighed 9 lb, 8 oz.

Sounds like a happy ending to a scary story? Well, not entirely.

While in the nursery, the baby turned out to have a bit of a limp hand. There is a great chance that it will pass within a few weeks or months, but there is also a chance that it will not. This is called Erb's palsy. Surely you've seen people with one hand a little bit shorter than the other, who can only partially use that hand? This is it.

Oh, I felt so bad when that delivery was over. Until the end of the shift, we discussed and debated the details of this birth. The more we discussed it, the more we realized that there was nothing we could have done to prevent it. These things just happen. But there are unanswered questions. Maybe if we had done an episiotomy, this wouldn't have happened? Maybe if she had not had an epidural, this wouldn't have happened? Maybe if we had offered her a C-section, this wouldn't have happened? And maybe if the mother had eaten less sugar while pregnant, and the baby had been a little smaller, this wouldn't have happened? Maybe, maybe, maybe…

By the way, in terms of studies that have been carried out on the subject, the answers to these questions are in dispute. The majority of cases of Erb's palsy occur before delivery. A Caesarean, for example, only reduces the risk of shoulder dystocia by half, not entirely.

And recently, a new study recommends not performing a preventive episiotomy. Shoulder dystocia also occurs in small babies, and even preterm babies, not just with large ones, and I know there's a link between epidurals and shoulder dystocia. In short, these questions are buzzing in my head like a hive of bothersome bees and my heart is full of emotions. I didn't want to cause harm to anyone, and what if it's something I could have prevented but didn't, and what will happen to this cute baby? Will she be okay? And what will I do when I meet this situation in the future, only without an instructor to take the matter into her hands at the critical moment… which would be the case, since I only have one more shift as a student?

Eitan said something that, believe it or not, eased my mind a little. The next day, when I was recounting my experience, he said, "Well, someone has to do this job." I responded, "Yes, but why me? It's really stressful!" So he replied, "You know that all people are part of this one big whole, like cells in a large body. So what does it matter if it's you or someone else that gets stressed about something? It's like preferring that your right hand is scratched instead of your left."

I do not know if it translates well in writing, but to me it was very helpful. And here I still am, and I can see now that events like these are just part of this special profession I have chosen for myself, and I have to learn to cope with them.

Meanwhile, I am sending that cute baby good thoughts and wishes for her wellbeing.

Apparently you can learn homeopathy, Chinese medicine, and Shiatsu in one day

Today we had a one-day course on the subject of alternative medicine, which was quite catastrophic for me. The lecturer was a bit arrogant and constantly said things that made me jump off my seat like, "**You've got** to do this and that..." or "Women **should** feel such and such..." as if there is only one way to deliver, only one way to give birth. And the high point for me was when she said, "I used to be like you, a midwife with a conventional medical approach." She does not know us, why does she think that she knows what our approach is?

Even without that, everything was highly superficial. "In order to increase contractions, you press here; to increase dilation, press here." In my eyes, this is being contemptuous toward Chinese medicine. It's as if someone would say, "Come and let us teach you Western medicine," and then give me a two-hour lecture and three hours to practice. "To remove a brain tumor, cut it out; to cure kidney cancer, apply chemotherapy." And then send us off to treat patients. Any tool, regardless of how efficient, can be dangerous if used without the appropriate background, knowledge and understanding of the whole system, including when it is advisable to use them, when it is not and so on.

I understand that the idea was to entice us to learn more about the subject, but not in this way. Besides, I have many doubts about the way alternative medicine is studied nowadays in Israel. Anyone who took a once or twice a week course for the span of a year, is considered a certified therapist with a diploma in a gilded frame to hang on their wall.

Eitan and I often discuss the fact that the more time something requires in order to become proficient in it, the greater its value. Playing violin, for example, compared to playing the triangle. I believe that Chinese medicine should be learned for many years. In China, for example, a shiatsu course lasts four years and involves daily study and practice. How it is that in Israel one needs a lot less than that? Are we such experts in shiatsu?

My mother once almost died because of incorrect use of alternative medicine; not because it did not work, but because it did. The treatment took care of the symptoms, but not the disease, which was left to rage on, unchecked.

Well, as you can see, I'm a little fired up. There were other things that annoyed me, but the time allocated for my complaints is already spent...

The truth is that I think my being angry is related to something else, actually. I just came back from the post office in Tel Aviv, where I paid the final installment for the course. Behind me in line was a man with Erb's palsy. I still think a lot about the baby from last week and I discussed this with my course coordinator, a conversation that helped put things in perspective. She told me about her incidents with severe shoulder dystocia and what happened. What eases me about all these conversations is that every midwife I talk to about the subject tells me that only on very few occasions did shoulder dystocia result in paralysis of the baby. These rare cases are so traumatic, however, that they remember every detail of every single one of these births.

Midwife proposes... God disposes

This should have been a day that helped me recover from the dreadful birth with the shoulder dystocia I told you about. It should have been a day when I was given at least two natural births, which went smoothly – perhaps some woman delivering her fifth child, who arrived at reception fully dilated; and another who was giving birth for the second time and wanted to deliver in the birth chair. Something nice and healthy like that, without complications, to complete my internship. But in reality, as usual, everything that could go wrong did go wrong.

It started in the morning. We arrived for our shift and there was a lovely woman who was trying to have a VBAC.[27] That is, to have a vaginal birth after her previous child was born by C-section. She

---

27 VBAC – Vaginal Birth After Caesarean. The notion used to be that once you had a Caesarean you can never go back. In fact women were once not allowed to try and give birth vaginally after a Caesarean out of fear that the scar over the uterus would not stand the pressure of contractions and the uterus would rupture; a very dangerous situation for the mother and her child. But in recent years, there have been more and more studies showing that the chance of uterine rupture in a VBAC is relatively low – about 0.7%. If the woman has already given birth vaginally after the surgery, the chance of rupture drops even lower. However there are interventions that are not recommended in a VBAC, such as aggressive labor induction, and there are situations that require careful evaluation, such as the delivery of a big baby or that of twins. The chances of a successful VBAC depend on many factors, including the cause of the Caesarean section in the past, fetal weight, etc. On average, there is about 70% success rate, although this also depends on the policy of the hospital in which the birth is taking place. And despite all that, the most common reason for a C-section is a previous C-section.

had been fully dilated for half an hour and was pushing. Throughout the birth, there were severe decelerations in the FHR and every passing moment the situation looked worse. After an hour, we had no choice. The doctor still tried to make a failed attempt to pull the baby by vacuum, but within fifteen minutes the baby was born by C-section, with an Apgar score of 4/8[28], meaning not good. The umbilical cord was wrapped tightly around his neck three times, and his amniotic fluid had meconium.

This was a bad start. Half an hour later, the same thing happened, only with another woman: heart rate decelerations without recovery between contractions, meconium liquor and an emergency C-section.

Then came a woman whom I thought would be my savior. She was about to give birth for the fourth time; a real Jedi and a lovely woman to whom I immediately felt connected, despite our different backgrounds. We spent the entire shift together. At first, everything

---

28 Apgar score - when the baby is born, the midwife or doctor will assess the extent of the baby's adjustment to life outside the womb and the extent of the baby's need for help, such as providing oxygen, airway suctioning or even full resuscitation. In order to create uniformity and clarity, the baby is assessed according to several criteria, including color, breathing, response to stimulus, pulse and muscle tone. Every baby is assessed at one minute after birth and again after five minutes. If necessary, a further Apgar score can be calculated at ten minutes after birth. Evaluation is done almost automatically by the midwife and does not require special tests. For example, a baby who, one minute after being born, is crying well and waving his arms, and whose color is rapidly becoming a paintbrush pink, will get an Apgar score of 9. If after five minutes the color has become all pink, the second score will be a 10. A low Apgar score may be caused by congenital disease of the newborn, events that occurred during the delivery or medications that the mother received during labor. Apgar scores at birth have no high predictive power of the baby's future state, and there may be babies with low Apgar scores whose development will be completely normal.

seemed great: the monitor was great, she spent a lot of time in the shower and she even walked outside a little.

Now, are you by any chance familiar with the Rule of Threes? A doctor once told me that if two women bled dangerously during her shift, then surely a third was destined to arrive with the same problem. It sounds like superstition, but I've seen medical decisions that were taken based on a fear of bad luck.

Anyway, let us return to the woman's story. Within an hour, her water broke and it contained meconium. Then there was a severe deceleration in the FHR that didn't recover. After a while, the pulse did recover but there were further decelerations. Then the delivery didn't progress at all for several hours. We prepared her for surgery, just to be on the safe side, and at the same time tried to convince her that she still doesn't need surgery, a strange situation. Ultimately, she did give birth vaginally, to the joy of everyone!

In the delivery room, there was another woman with meconium liquor and decelerations in pulse. When I called, she was just coming out of her C-section ... Oh, and there was another woman, with Meconial water (of course), who had frightening heart beat decelerations and who eventually gave birth after being induced.

Sometimes you just have one of those days, and everyone is really frustrated by it. After a day like this, I feel like some sort of technician, who just spends her whole day hooking up external and internal monitors,[29] taking blood tests, giving inductions and record-

29 Internal monitoring – with most births, the fetal monitor is put on the woman's abdomen. Sometimes, when the external monitor is not receiving a good signal from the baby's heart, due to its position or due to the abdominal wall being very thick, an electrode is put directly onto the baby's head. That is called internal monitoring. Internal monitoring is also used in the birth of twins, when an internal monitor is hooked up to the first twin and an external monitor is connected to the second, in order to avoid a situation in which only one baby is being monitored.

ing everything she does on five different forms, chasing the doctor to come and see the monitor and so on. And the work phase spectrum ranges between emergency situations and short moments of relaxation: "Oh, there is fetal bradycardia: **connect to oxygen! Lie on your left side! Give her an IV! Call a doctor!**"... "Oh, there is a decrease in blood pressure! **Call the anesthesiologist! Give her an IV! Take blood tests!**" And in the midst of all this, there's the family and the woman giving birth, and they hear every word the staff says and get anxious, looking around and trying to figure out what the facial expression of their doctor or midwife means, asking repeatedly if everything is okay and if it wouldn't be better to just go to surgery. And I find myself torn between the desire not to stress them, since stress itself stops the delivery, and the desire to tell the whole truth and nothing but the truth. After all, they need to know the truth of the situation in order to make the decision that is right for them.

Let's say I examine a woman and see that her dilation hasn't progressed at all in two hours. The woman looks at me full of hope and wants to hear that there is a dilation of 7 centimeters and I tell her that there is still only a dilation of two and a half centimeters. Many women get really desperate in those kinds of situations. So what to do? Tell her that there might be a little more shortening of the cervix now? Maybe that the head has descended a little? I always try to find something positive to say. And often, just then, the doctor comes in and says, "So? It hasn't progressed at all in the last hour, eh?" And he turns to the woman and says, "Your birth is a little stuck, huh?"

In general, the whole idea of vaginal examinations is very much connected to Western medicine's way of thinking; the need to know exactly, at every stage, where the baby is, what the dilation is, how short the cervix is, what is the time between contractions and so on. There's even a new machine that does it. You place it in the vagina at the beginning of birth, and you can see everything that goes on in there, live on cable television. The next step will probably be to connect a fetal monitor to every woman from the moment of conception... Big Brother sees everything.

The concept of 'active management of labor' says that you must track the progress of birth and when the rate of progress is not as expected, you must start induction by breaking the waters or providing IV Pitocin. According to proponents of this approach, this prevents the need for surgery (ha!) and birth complications (ha, ha, ha!). The thing is that the "expected rate of progress" was determined decades ago by a man named Friedman, who collected data on fewer than a hundred births. Today he wouldn't have dared to publish his results in any medical magazine, and yet the system still acts according to his conclusions.

Sometimes, it is important to check the dilation, for example, to determine when a woman should push. This is highly relevant when an epidural has been administered and, by the way, once you have already had an intervention, such as an epidural, other interventions become necessary, because often the birth will not progress without induction, but that's another story.

In principle, a woman should feel the need to push and not have to wait for the green light of "fully dilated." But, many women feel the need to push, and do, right from the start with a dilation of 2 centimeters. This can tear the cervix or cause edema, which will later cause complications in the delivery.

There are women who push when at a dilation of 8 to 9 centimeters, and a number of homebirth midwives I met at a conference in Germany said that there is nothing wrong with this, as long as the woman feels she has to push. Our human body is very intelligent. It can be a good idea to listen to it from time to time.

Another reason to check dilation is that it can help in making a decision when something goes wrong - for example, when there is a sudden, severe deceleration in the pulse that does not recover between contractions. Such a situation can cause permanent damage to the fetus within minutes. The question is what to do next: go straight to surgery, try to pull the baby out by vacuum or simply tell the woman to push and that's it. So if, for example, she has a dilation of 3 centimeters, it is clear that you must go straight to surgery.

There are also women who want to be examined in order to know how much they have progressed; while at other times, it's just the curiosity of the midwife.

But above all, in an ordinary natural birth, there is no reason to check for dilation, and to support this claim are the millions of zebras, cats, apes, dogs, hamsters, giraffes, elephants, cows and horses who give birth without anyone checking their dilation. Hmm… I wonder what would be considered full dilation in an elephant…

So that was my day. At the end we decided, Michal and I, that there was no way that this would be my last day of internship. It just couldn't be. We decided that I would come back again the next week.

Back in the monastery

Imagine that I, a midwifery student, am sitting in the nurses' station; in the room next to me, there's a delivery; I have nothing better to do, and still I choose not to go in to see it.

When I think about it I can't believe it myself. I, who wanted to attend every delivery I possibly could, and stayed sometimes seven hours after my shift, just to be in one...

But on this day, I stayed put, trying to curl into a ball in my chair, with no success. The shift supervisor urged me, "Don't you want to come and see it? You can learn something from observing too."

Sure, I thought to myself, you can mostly learn how **not** to deliver.

Oh well, reluctantly I went and watched as the midwife told the weary woman, "*Shidi, shidi*" which is Arabic for "Push, push." After a minute, her tired and indifferent tone disappeared and was replaced by shouting. The midwife shouted at the woman not to recoil every time she put her hand in her vagina. Later she moved on to threats, "If you don't stay still, I'll cut you!" Then the midwife inserted both hands into the woman's vagina in order to stretch it, or at least that's what she thought she was doing. Now you have to understand, it's not that the birth wasn't progressing or something. It was a quick delivery, and the woman gave birth fifteen minutes after getting to the delivery room.

Another dose of "*shidi, shidi*" and "don't move," and the woman started to cry. Then the nursing assistant entered and started pushing on the woman's belly. I immediately told her to stop, and she did, but I know that they ask her to do that in the rest of the deliveries here. In other hospitals, this is a medical procedure that was stopped a long time ago, because it endangers women and can cause internal bleeding.

When the baby was born, the midwife put him on the woman's tummy, just long enough for her to cut the umbilical cord, and then he was taken to be weighed and was given some eye ointment. Then he was taken to the nursery. Doesn't anyone find it jarring or strange that the mother, who waited nine months to see her baby, saw him for just thirty seconds and then it was bye, bye?

Then it was the placenta's turn. Did you really think it would escape violent intervention with that? No way! Not if it doesn't want to come out in twenty seconds. In this case, you press on the belly, massage the uterus and tug on the umbilical cord. That's how you make things go faster so you can go and have your coffee and a cigarette. Sometimes the uterus comes out with it... Oh well, never mind. Don't make a fuss, that's very rare.[30]

---

30 A few words about how long it takes for the placenta to be born. The placenta should be born a short while after the baby leaves the uterus. Until the placenta is out, the uterus cannot contract. Uterine contraction is actually a mechanism that prevents fatal bleeding after delivery. In most cases, there's no bleeding until the placenta comes out, because the placenta is still attached to the uterine wall. Once it separates from the uterine wall, it usually comes out. This is a natural process that often happens within minutes but can sometimes take longer. Just yesterday, a friend of mine, a homebirth midwife in London, told me that she had a birth where the placenta separated only after three hours. Since the woman wasn't bleeding, there was no reason to try and speed up the process, at least not in a home birth. If the woman had been bleeding, it could have been, as mentioned, a life-threatening condition, and then she would have had to intervene. In hospitals, there is no time to wait for an hour or two or three for the placenta to come out. The room must be cleared for the next mother, and in addition, until the placenta comes out, the woman is at risk, because, as I said, dangerous bleeding may occur due to partial separation, so the midwife has to be with the woman at all times. Since the midwife usually handles two or three women at the same time, it is impossible to wait forever. Each hospital has its own protocol for when to intervene. Some hospitals wait for half an hour, some an hour, and

After the placenta came out, they put the bed back together, injected Pitocin to prevent bleeding and bye, bye. The midwife left the delivery room. She had done her part.

That is it. The good old days of my internship were gone and now I was back at the hospital where I worked, a hospital I ended up in from lack of choice, as there were no job openings for midwives anywhere else. It was a rude awakening from my romantic fantasy about how interesting and unique it might be to work in a place like this, which is half hospital, half monastery. I have always liked the movie *The Sound of Music* and as a child I found that there was something about monasteries that attracted and compelled me. Yet despite the unusual nature of the place, which made me feel like I was living in a different world, or maybe a different universe, there was little pleasure to being there, and it was hard to believe that

---

some more; if the woman is bleeding, then you do not wait at all and rightly so. When the placenta doesn't separate, a doctor inserts, usually under general anesthesia (if there is no epidural), his hand into the uterus and peels the placenta out. Then he checks that no pieces were left inside. This procedure is often accompanied by antibiotics to prevent infection of the uterus. This action is performed even if the placenta came out but there is still suspicion that parts of it remained inside. Pressing on the woman's belly is a controversial action. The naturalistic approach claims there is no need to press after the delivery, but that one should give the placenta time to separate and be born on its own. Pressing does stimulate the separation, but there are risks: it can cause only part of the placenta to separate, it can cause uncoordinated contraction of the uterus, and it can (in combination with pulling the umbilical cord) cause a reversal of the womb which means that the uterus comes out of the vagina. It is a life-threatening condition and may result in loss of the uterus. Besides, pressing on the belly is also very painful for the woman. There are more natural ways to speed up placenta separation, such as placing the baby on the mother, creating a peaceful environment with dim light, allowing eye contact between mother and baby, breastfeeding, warming up the room and the woman - all of which increase the secretion of oxytocin in the woman's brain.

only a few kilometers separated our delivery room from the one where I had experienced my memorable internship.

But back to our story… so what did I learn from this birth?

I learned how I didn't want to behave towards women in labor, how I don't want to deliver a baby, what I don't want the first minutes after a birth to look like and the kind of midwife I never want to be like. But all these things I already knew before. So basically I didn't learn anything new, because I witnessed this scene, with minor changes, with different midwives every day – of course not all of them, there are some righteous men in Sodom. I didn't learn anything and I only felt sadness, frustration and pain.

After the midwife had gone away to write a report on the birth and I stayed behind, alone with the woman, the room echoed with emptiness. A moment ago a birth had taken place here; passionate, painful and real. And now, just five minutes later, there was no trace of what had happened, and no baby. There was only a woman lying down with a pad between her legs and an IV drip attached to her hand. I wanted to comfort her, but didn't know what to say. What should I say? Maybe something like, "Well, we're finished. You can go to sleep now."

When Zona met Corona

"*The egg is surrounded by a layer of Zona-pellucida but also a layer of granulosa cells, called cumulus oophorus, which form the egg follicle wall. The corona radiata also consists of cumulus cells. The stem that holds the eggs is called the corpus cumulus.*"

I'm studying for my certification exam and I find myself reading this paragraph over and over without understanding any of it. I don't know why... I don't usually think anatomy is boring, and when there is a lesson about physiology I totally melt. The human body is simply a wonderful masterpiece, and the way things work ranges from the unbelievable to the impossible.

I remember that our anatomy teacher at nursing school told us about someone who became religious after he learned how the Henle Loop in the kidney works. It is very complicated but simply amazing. That person just realized that something that miraculous could not have formed by accident and that there must be someone who designed it.

I think that our bodies can teach us a lot. If only we could be as harmonious as our bodies; if we could make the right choices like intestinal epithelial cells; if we could only get rid of all that is undesirable like nephrons in the kidneys; if we could only be as dedicated and persistent as our hearts. These qualities live in us, if we know where to look, so it is so extraordinary to me to learn all this.

Well, I got a bit carried away. This is what happens when I study for an exam for several weeks straight.

I already feel quite ready for the exam, and I don't think this coming week will make me more prepared than I already am. Anyway, I'm on vacation until the exam, so I get up every day at eleven, walk the dog, do some reading. This week I read *Harry Potter and the Deathly Hallows*, *Kensuke's Kingdom* and *Shadow of the Giant*. Not bad for someone who's supposed to study all day... don't tell my course coordinator, though.

Today I actually studied hard. I study most of the time while walking the streets of my village, because otherwise I fall asleep within two minutes. Occasionally a friend calls me with a pressing question, such as "during vaginal examination, you feel the front fontanel[31] at six o'clock. Which position is the baby in?" I want this to be behind me so badly. I've been studying for five years in a row - first nursing, then a bachelor's degree and now midwifery; and I always have the lingering feeling that there is some coursework to submit or a test to study for. I want to be free from it.

Well, I'm going to read a little about disseminated intravascular coagulation...

31 In the baby's skull, there are two openings, called fontanels, which close during the first two years of its life. During vaginal examination, you can feel them and figure out in what position the baby is lying; for example, an occipital posterior position or face presentation. Determining the baby's posture helps the midwife decide how to change a woman's position, in trying to resolve a lack of progress in birth, which could be caused by how the baby entered the birth canal.

Three months later

I come home, turn on the computer, enter my ID number and test number...

Score: 86 percent.

I'm a midwife.

I'm a midwife?

I'M A MIDWIFE!!!!!!!!!!!!!!!

Jumping into deep waters

Today I attended three births: three women, two baby boys and one baby girl. This is my output in my first day as a certified midwife. Not bad, eh?

When my head nurse talked to us, the two new midwives in the ward, about our orientation for the job, she said that we would start with three weeks in reception, and only then would we move on to the delivery room. As it turned out, however, I found myself in the delivery room during my first day of orientation, and I received my first birth at 3:20 PM – twenty minutes after the start of my shift. Oh well, I shouldn't be surprised. Hospitals may be chock full of intelligible words and intellectual minds, but they often lack good sound judgment.

In theory, it should have been a pleasant experience. The woman was giving birth for the third time, she was progressing really fast, she hadn't been given any analgesic or induction and the procedure didn't call for an episiotomy. In practice, things were a little different. My head nurse was with me and at some point, as the woman pushed, she shoved me aside, stuck both hands - eight fingers total - into the woman's vagina and started shouting at her, even though there was no reason to do so. I think, though I'm not sure, she gave her a small tear in the perineum. After the baby's head was out, she pushed me aside again and delivered the baby's body. I waited patiently for the placenta but after a minute she got tired of waiting and began to press on the woman's belly and told me in a condescending tone, "Someday you'll start to learn from us, as we all learn from one another."

The woman screamed in pain, which was caused by the pressure on the abdomen, and then the placenta came out. Meanwhile, the baby was wrapped up, presented to the family and transferred to the orientation center. Ah, sorry, I meant the nursery.

Welcome to our hospital. This (or worse) is the way of most of our births. Any attempt to do things differently rewards me with glares of contempt, gossip about me behind my back and shouting by the midwife and/or doctor. It is a horrible place but this is all I have until a vacancy opens up at the hospital where I did my internship… which probably won't happen for at least a few years.

Within this situation, I mean to try and do everything I can to navigate and do what I believe is right. It means, for example, at least initially, to argue less (the goal is not to argue at all, but I don't think I'll succeed there) and to perform an episiotomy on every woman giving birth for the first time, for a few months at least, so that later I can decide with whom I can act freely and with whom I cannot. Will I survive such a period without forgetting who I am and what I really believe in? Here, I found another reason for writing this diary: to remember who I am and who I want to be.

The second birth I attended was nicer. Miriam, the head nurse, who had stayed since the morning shift, had gone home and left me in the hands of Ruba, who has been a midwife for several years now and is one of the few who actually treat women nicely here. Ruba has a charming personality and a fascinating life story. She emigrated from Jordan, is smart, highly educated, creative and very confident, and I was happy to be with her.

The woman was giving birth for the first time, with an epidural and an 8-centimeter dilation. The monitor showed everything to be normal; the woman pushed in the right way; and ultimately she gave birth to a beautiful baby girl who weighed 8 lb, 4 oz.

I had given her an episiotomy, which Ruba said was very elegant; what a strange thing to say about a woman's vaginal cut. The doctor said it was a little too close to the rectum. I wanted to say that it was unnecessary, but nobody asked me. Anyway, I should work on the direction of my incisions. In the end, I will be an episiotomy expert, and this is an important skill to have. The truth is that during my internship I did only maybe four or five of those, so surely I have something to learn here.

The third birth was the icing on the cake: a lovely woman, on her sixth birth, who arrived with a 5 centimeter dilation and gave birth within an hour. Unfortunately, while I went to the bathroom, Ruba gave her Demerol,[32] which is almost mandatory in our hospital, because if not it could have been a delivery with only minimal intervention. No one entered the room and she didn't really need a midwife to give birth. The baby just slipped out, a tiny thing that weighed just 6 pounds.

I am also getting better at hooking up an IV drip port - and not just into a vein in the crook of the elbow, where it is not a big deal, but also in the back of the hand and forearm. Apart from that, today I learned how to file everything in at least five different places. Long live bureaucracy!

I feel a little emotionally detached from these births. Births are seen here as something very technical: the baby is inside; the baby needs to come out. The thought that a woman would like to see,

---

32 Demerol is a drug from the opioids family that is given to women in childbirth for pain relief. Demerol causes drowsiness and relieves some pain. Since one of its side effects is nausea, it should be combined with an anti-nausea medication such as Phenergan, hence the nickname 'cocktail'. Other side effects are dizziness and confusion. Many women report that since they were asleep between contractions and woke up only during them, they experienced the birth as one endless stream of ongoing pain. However, for some women, Demerol is a welcome relief from the pain of contractions; for example, women who have a long latent phase with no progress in dilation. Demerol also enables relaxation, which often allows for a speedier birth. The drug passes easily through the placenta to the fetus and may cause the baby to be drowsy at birth and may even cause respiratory and breastfeeding difficulties. Since the mother is still drowsy at the time of birth, it may hinder the initial bonding between the mother and her baby.

hug or even breastfeed her baby is probably considered strange among the medical team here. Otherwise, why do they remove the baby straight away, before the mother can touch him and look him in the eyes? And in truth, I think most women here probably see it the same way, because most of them don't want to see the baby and when you ask them they say, "Take it." This is what happens when they are given Demerol, in most cases.

But not all is lost. There is definitely room for small changes, especially during the night and evening shifts, when there isn't a battalion of consultants looking over my shoulder - or worse still - pressing on the woman's abdomen and pushing their hands into her vagina.

Tomorrow I have another evening shift, in the delivery room or maybe in reception this time... I guess I should go to bed already. Goodnight.

Juggling whilst running

I just came back from perhaps the most difficult evening shift I have ever had. Because of the rush, I didn't work as a midwife but as a nurse. It also turned out that I was not supposed to start attending births until I receive my license in the mail. During the shift, I took care of seven women who had undergone C-sections, a few more women whose waters had broken, women in the latent stage and women who had to be under supervision due to all kinds of pregnancy problems. We had an emergency C-section because of a full placental abruption – thank God, the baby is fine - two urgent D&C's because of incomplete abortions and heavy bleeding, and a woman with severe preeclampsia who, while pushing during labor, began to bleed from her ear. Due to the fear of brain injury, and all kinds of other horrible scenarios that you can imagine, we urgently delivered the baby by vacuum. Besides all that, there were two births and a few more pregnant women with abdominal or side pain; all this with a total of four team members.

Never have I run so much from one side of the ward to the other, while carrying an IV bag/towel/robe/pain relief injections/surgery consent form to be signed by the woman/trays/glasses of water and much more.

In addition, each woman had five to ten family members with her, who gathered at the door and kept demanding to know when she would give birth. One of them was completely drunk and it turns out that he almost gave me a beating. Luckily I wasn't aware of that and so I wasn't scared and didn't panic. I was informed of it only later.

These kinds of shifts scare me so much. The stress reaches unbelievable levels, and at any given time you have ten things to do and three distractions. Let's say, you have to record that you gave the woman a painkiller. It's very important. They are included in the list of "dangerous drugs" and we have to be very meticulous in recording them. At the same time, another woman who had a C-section wants you to give her something for the pain; on your way to the nurses' station, someone wants to ask you something, while another husband asks for a towel for his wife; Suddenly, two phones and the call light in the delivery room all sound at the same time; another woman suddenly comes to the reception desk and cries about a terrible headache she has - God forbid it might be preeclampsia, just don't start to convulse on me now – and then the husband who asked for the towel demands to know why can't he have his towel. Wait a moment! What about the drug recording?

And so it goes on, and in all this mess I am afraid to make a mistake, give the wrong drug to someone, forget to record something important (although, by the way, we also get chewed out for unimportant things we forget to record). These errors can cost lives, or, at best, only my license as a nurse or midwife.

Someone once told me that, in the United States, the quota is three patients at most per nurse, and if a nurse happens to go over her quota (say four or five patients), it is recorded. This way, if she makes a mistake, she is not liable to be sued. Not to mention that nurses there almost never give drugs; this is done by pharmacists. They do not take blood pressure and temperature, and they certainly do not make beds or serve food. They mainly counsel and explain, which is the most important thing one can do, really. They manage care and make sure that everything that needs to be done is done; they oversee the big picture regarding the condition of the patient and don't run around like a clockwork monkey. Today I felt like someone trying to juggle twelve balls at the same time, with balls falling down from every direction.

But we're here and not in the United States. And they also have their problems, such as, despite the fact that there are plenty of human resources, many people have no money to pay for treatment and get stuck in public hospitals, which are not really that good. Each system has its advantages and disadvantages, but despite that, I feel that working as we did today really crossed the line.

Death visited the delivery room again this week

During the morning shift, a couple came into the waiting room. The man seemed impatient and restless and the woman was anxious and nervous. It turned out that for the past five days, she had not felt any movements at all from the fetus and so she finally went to a family health center, which referred her to the ER. My first instinct was to ask, "Why [the hell] did you come only now? Why did you wait?" But I knew that if the worst did come true, I did not want to add any more to this woman's inflated cup of guilt. Besides, if I had been in her shoes, am I sure I would have acted differently? I can understand the fear of bad news and the desire and need to delay it a little longer; to draw out the hope as long as possible.

I admitted the woman, who turned out to be in week twenty-six, and tried to find a pulse with the monitor. I was reminded of the words of my course instructor, as she said, for the umpteenth time, "When a woman enters the delivery room, the first thing you do is to check the FHR." So I looked for a pulse, and at first we heard one: boom, stillness, stillness, boom... The woman burst into tears of relief and told me she thought the baby was dead. I wasn't at all sure if it was the baby's heart rate or the woman's, so I tried to look for a continuous pulse and not only a beat here and there. A fetal monitor, after all, is not really the pinnacle of accuracy.

After a few minutes, I called the doctor, who tried and could not find a pulse. He called for a more senior doctor and showed him the ultrasound image. There was no pulse.

Now the doctor had to tell the woman what was going on. I have heard many terrible stories about the ways in which doctors deliver such information to women, and I've witnessed some examples myself. I was afraid of how this doctor would break the news. He chose a very gradual and puzzling way:

Doctor: "Look, there is a problem with your baby. We think he is not entirely okay."

Woman: "What do you mean?"

Doctor: "He doesn't feel so well."

Woman: "What do you mean?"

Doctor: "There is a problem with his breathing. He is not breathing so well. He really does not breathe at all. And he also has a problem with his heart. He has no pulse. In fact, you could say he is not alive."

I do not know. What do you think about this way? On the one hand, it is good to give bad news gradually and certainly good that he told her the fetus was "not alive" and not just that "he has no pulse" or something ambiguous like that. Many women, when told there is no pulse, do not understand that the fetus is in fact dead. But this whole thing of going from "doesn't feel so well" to "is not alive" felt just weird; almost ridiculous. It would be more appropriate to say something like, "I have bad news for you" and then continue from there.

The woman cried after she realized what had happened, and I was glad to see that the doctors were sensitive and gave her the time and space she needed to figure things out. When her husband came and heard the news, he responded in the most masculine way possible. He mustered all his might and main, took a deep breath, and said, "Okay. So what do we do now? How can I help? How do we get this over with as quickly as possible? What are you going to do to her now? Who will look after her? Can you personally make sure that she gets the best treatment as quickly as possible?"

He had to do something about this terrible helplessness; had to turn their pain into action. He said, "I want her to give birth so we can go home and be done with it." I talked to him a little bit and I tried to make him understand that even after she delivers, they will not be "done with it" but only at the beginning of a long road to recovery, and that it is okay to grieve, to hurt, and not instantly carry on as if nothing has happened.

Then we got her hospitalized, with all the necessary bureaucracy, which is so burdensome and unnecessary at such a time. We had to ask all kinds of questions take blood tests and sign forms. It's too bad we cannot skip this step. I accompanied her to her room and we hugged and during this whole time she was crying.

And now what? We had to induce labor somehow. For some reason, over the last two weeks we had had many cases of intrauterine fetal demise, and all of these women had a few nerve wracking days, while the staff tried to induce labor in all kinds of ways. Usually it takes a few days until they succeed, during which the woman and her family have a very difficult time - especially the husband, who feels, as I said, extremely helpless in the face of a reality he cannot change, cannot reverse.

This woman was a bit more fortunate, and when I came the next day to the evening shift she had already delivered. She gave birth to a baby girl who had six fingers on each hand and several other birth defects that apparently were the cause of her death. The couple refused an autopsy and preferred to bury her. By the way, this is a custom I respect in Arab society. They name and bury the stillborn babies, unlike Jews, who usually do not take the stillborn child with them. I think that when the baby has a name and you can visit the grave, it becomes a part of the family and not some nameless secret ghost that you cannot talk about and cannot reminisce about or shed tears over.

I went to talk to her a bit and we had a good conversation. She was very open about everything and told me how she felt yesterday before coming to the hospital, and how she felt when she realized the baby was dead, and that at the time of birth she still hoped it was a mistake and that maybe the baby would be born alive. She talked about herself, about how difficult her first delivery was and how despite that she wasn't afraid of this pregnancy. She really wanted a daughter and had been very happy she was about to give birth to a baby girl. She also talked about her family. It turns out that her sister-in-law had undergone the same thing two weeks earlier, and that her cousin had a son who died at the age of two months. "God takes his favorites to him," she said.

We talked about the fact that although "it is better that it happened this way" as opposed to the possibility of having a baby with severe deformities, and that "all is from Allah" and "there is nothing you can do" and "*Inshallah,*[33] you will soon become pregnant again and give birth to a healthy baby"; yet it still hurts and it's okay that it hurts. I told her that in fact almost every woman goes through at least one miscarriage in her life and many women experience late miscarriages or still births, but they hardly talk about it, so it's as if it didn't happen. We agreed that it is part of life, but still, it hurts.

Later, the family came to visit and they called me over. They offered me chocolate and showed me their son, ten months old, chubby and cute, with round cheeks and big eyes. It felt special, to enter into the life of a family, if only for one day. But what a day it was! And I am glad to know just how meaningful they were for me and how meaningful I was for them, and that even if the relationship does not continue in any apparent way, it is recorded somewhere… it exists.

Most medical personnel are reluctant to deal with women having a stillbirth. I think some of that fear of death is really associated with our sense of failure as a medical team; the fact that we were unable to prevent the death. Or maybe it's our own fear of mortality that becomes more tangible every time we witness a death.

I learn so much from these women. I feel that with every such sad case I encounter, I have more to give to these women, more ways to help and more ways to support. I begin to understand the

33 With the help of God (Arabic).

meaning of accumulated experience, of theory becoming fact. It all adds up to a broader spectrum of knowledge: feelings, notions, words that can and cannot be used, touch, glances, cries and consolations. Information accumulates in me like in a computer, and gets filed away, ready to be retrieved and used at a later time.

I am not afraid of death. It is so clear to me that man is not his mortal body but something much higher, something that lives in a body it has borrowed for only a few years. I believed in it even before I was a nurse, but my experience as a nurse has turned this theoretical faith into something completely tangible.

To see a man whose body is an absolute wreck, and to hear him speak as a young man full of vigor... to see the spark of life in a person's eyes suddenly disappear... that person is "dead" but his body is still there, as if someone is just not home anymore. To hear my good friend who was dying tell of his experiences on the other side, which he visited several times before he passed on and from where something or someone came several times to visit, help and prepare him to acclimatize to the other side.

My friend said, "Don't be sad. Where I'm going is much better and much more beautiful than here." The encounter with the wisdom that came to him when he was on the threshold between the two worlds, the tranquility that surrounded him, and the feeling in the room where he lay in his house, was the most incredible experience of my life so far.

I'm not afraid to die, but my body is afraid of dying, so it is cautious when driving and when approaching the edge of a cliff on a hike, and it is horrified when it thinks something is threatening it such as chest pains or something similar. But the body is not the highest part of us, and it is our choice in which part to reside most of the time.

I am not afraid of death, but rather see it as a great adventure; the beginning of what is really important - of real life, after we have gathered a little bit of experience. A person must have a body in order to grow and develop, since in the spiritual world there is no difficulty, no hardship; only the material world can provide the necessary hardships for growth. It's like lifting weights in order to develop one's muscles. It is impossible to develop muscles in space, where there is no resistance.

And death is really a friend; the great liberator.

The tear is not important
Let it go, do not be scared.
What is important is the eye
That looks to the future.

The tear grows and curves,
Pregnant with sorrow.
Bear it
And let it slide away.

Do not hold it,
Let it go.

A beautiful birth along the way

A young, smiling woman with a sweet face came in to give birth to her first baby. For some reason she was not accompanied by anyone, so I tried to be with her as much as possible. One of the things that set her apart was her openness. She asked for an epidural, which is very, very rare in our hospital, and thus was spared the usual dose of analgesic given to almost every woman that gives birth here. She was good-spirited and cheerful, or as a friend of mine would put it, a real "good egg."

Just before the baby was born, her contractions suddenly stopped. So I suggested she try giving herself a nipple massage. Massaging the nipples causes the pituitary gland to release oxytocin, the hormone that causes contractions. Such suggestions typically get embarrassed responses in our hospital. Very few women will agree to try it, and even then it would have to be done through a shirt and a blanket, in a closed room, alone and in the dark. This woman, however, raised her shirt and started rubbing vigorously.

"It really helps!" she announced happily. Then she grabbed my hand and put it on her belly and told me, "Put your hand here, it helps me!" So I put it there and it really helped.

We told her that she had done well and that soon the baby will be out, and she said, "Excellent! Encourage me more. Tell me what good progress we're making and how great I am!" So we told her just that and the delivery went along well.

Then she gave birth to a baby weighing eight and a half pounds and was just thrilled about it. We were very happy too.

I'm finally, officially, a certified and registered midwife in the great State of Israel

A week ago, my long-awaited license finally arrived in the mail and now they're starting to put me to work not just as a nurse, but also as a midwife in the delivery room. It means that I do everything I did before, but now I am also attending births.

All these events were pushed a little to the side in my mind, since this was a very emotional week in our ward. An anesthesiologist who worked with us all the time, during Caesarean sections and epidurals (the operating room is right next to our ward and the doctors often come over for coffee, a cigarette or just small talk) was found dead in his car in the hospital parking lot, after taking his own life. The reason he did it is unknown and the entire hospital has been in turmoil for several days now. There are various conspiracy theories running around that try to explain why he did it; everything from an illicit affair to enormous debts. Someone even talked about the possibility of murder. It is strange that a trivial reason such as depression wasn't even mentioned, although it's the most common reason for suicide at his age. I guess it's not exciting enough.

He was a very nice man, the only one who was really kind to us, the midwives. Whatever it was that caused him to commit suicide, he did not share it with anyone, and this is a very lonely, desperate and sad thought.

In other news, we are in the midst of a heated dispute between the delivery room and maternity ward. Why isn't it possible to work together as friends, like human beings? Why must there be a competitive attitude or hostility everywhere? All you ever hear is, "We are making fewer mistakes than you," and "We work a lot harder than you!" As someone who has worked in both departments, I can say that wherever one goes, the work is hard and it always seems like one is working harder than others.

As part of this overall campaign, some very dramatic battles were fought today: there were bursts of crying; phones being slammed down to disconnect the other party; conversations with the hospital director; a whole lot of things done just out of spite, and a lot of, "We will show them not to mess with us!" Ugh.

Have I mentioned that my place of work is a monastery hospital for nuns? We have an abbess, who nags a little and annoys everyone most of the time. She speaks an incomprehensible blend of French-Arabic-Spanish and insists on conversing with us in this jumbled up dialect. Please try and imagine the following sentence with a heavy French accent, *"Min Hadi? Amalia? Sizarien? Shu fin Andha? Toxemia? Ooh la la..."*[34] There are also retired nuns and secondary nuns and a whole hierarchical structure that is very strange and that I do not pretend to understand, not even a little bit. Sometimes it seems that in order to reorganize the towel shelf and the sheet shelf we must get an approval from the Pope. I dream of the day when I write my novel or a hospital soap opera about a delivery room full of nuns. *Sister Margarita blushed under her white cap... "Dr. Samir! Are you taunting me?"* Something like that.

I admit that there are pleasant parts to this: a Christmas tree at Christmas; church bells ringing in the building next door; a Christmas present (a small floral porcelain elephant) from the old nun, Sister Mary Paul; the charming ancient architecture that includes an arched monastery courtyard, high ceilings, Jerusalem stone walls and a general feeling that is foreign to contemporary Israel.

---

34 Who is she? Oh, after surgery? What is the matter with her? She has toxemia? Ooh la la...

And there is also the diversity of the team. We have Jews, Muslims, Christians, Druze, doctors, nurses, midwives, the nursing assistants, the maintenance personnel and management. All are woven into an invisible but completely clear (not to me of course) system of hierarchy, respect, importance and so on. For a year and a half I puzzled my head over this question: who is higher on the ladder of importance here, a Muslim female doctor or a Jewish male doctor? One thing was crystal clear – the topmost rung was reserved for the Christian male doctors. A Jewish female midwife is somewhere in the middle, and the lowest rank is saved for a Jewish or Muslim cleaning woman.

I hope this didn't offend anyone; I know it's not very politically correct to say this. It would be nice to write that everybody loves everyone else and that peace, tranquility and equality prevail. But that's not how it works, and this invisible system of hierarchy is very rigid. It took me a year to realize that it even exists, and only now I understand why I was characterized as having a "slight communication problem." There are thousands of cultural nuances at play: the tone of voice you use, what you say and to whom and how and when. One could write a doctorate on this. I think that even today I only see the tip of the iceberg.

It's actually somewhat of a Middle Eastern microcosm, which is a bit depressing, because it makes me see what rifts we must bridge to establish real communication. Not only does each side fail to understand the other; each fails to understand that it doesn't understand. Add in the ordinary workplace politics: small intrigues, jealousy, love, friendships made and broken, complaints, the salary that is always too low, the conditions that are always inapt, the work schedule and annual leave, and "Why has no one ordered medium-sized sterile gloves if they ran out?" In the midst of this chaos, Dana received her license, so who cares? Sometimes I think that even I don't care... it looks like just another random thing that happened this week.

And yet, I received my license, and there are many cries of "*Mabruk*,[35] my friend" and I answer, "*Yibrach fichi*."[36] I've already attended two really nice births and two Caesareans. My hospital's approach is "just throw them in the water and they'll learn to swim." It was a little scary at first, but proved itself to work eventually. So today I had my first experience in the operating room and then attended a birth; treated a postpartum bleeding quite proficiently; forgot to fill in only three details on the birth chart; didn't fight with or get annoyed by anyone; and I started to like, really like, a midwife that I'd had quite a hard time with before, and it seemed to me that she started to like me too. I think this is a good start.

35 Congratulations (Arabic).

36 Bless you, too (Arabic).

Truck engines and babies

Today I attended a birth. The mother-to-be was a beautiful woman, giving birth for the first time. She had depths I'm not used to seeing. As a child, she underwent surgery for a brain tumor and it changed her worldview as well as her sense of self. For some reason, I felt a bit like her sister or best friend. Later on, her husband said to me, "You know you two look alike?"

She arrived in the morning, and during her examination I found she was 3 centimeters dilated. After being admitted, she walked around the contraction room until noon. Then she came up to me and told me she thought I should examine her again. I did, and she was 7 centimeters dilated. So she stayed in the delivery room and we connected a monitor. The FHR wasn't the best, but there was no strong indication that intervention was needed. The woman asked for an analgesic and received one, and so she slept between contractions until she was fully dilated. Despite the analgesic, she was charming and not as dazed as one might expect. She smiled most of the time and was very calm.

She told me, "Since I had my experience, I always see God in front of me, in everything I do, and I'm not afraid."

Her husband, who in the meantime had come from work and joined us, was very excited and very loving. He tried to explain that he could read the fetal monitor because the noise an engine makes and the sound of the monitor are similar, at least in principle, and as a truck driver he's supposed to be attentive to such noises and understand their meaning. In any other situation this might have sounded ridiculous, but somehow, at that time, it sounded perfectly reasonable.

When she was fully dilated, there were two tiny decelerations in the pulse on the monitor; nothing drastic, but I called a doctor just to be on the safe side, especially since I'm new. Since there were no other women in the delivery room, and no one had anything to do, two midwives, a doctor and an assistant joined us. The room wasn't very large and there were a lot of people in there, but they were quiet and did not disturb us.

The midwife who was supervising me told me to perform an episiotomy, but she was not particularly assertive, and in my opinion the perineum was very flexible. Besides, the doctor who was with us was really charming and not the kind who shouts, "Why didn't you do an episiotomy?" So I decided not to make an incision, despite the fact that the fetus was estimated to weigh 8 lb, 3 oz.

The woman pushed just the way she should, and at one point, half the head was out, but just half. Then she asked for water, and there was no contraction for a few minutes, and it was a little funny to see a woman with half a head peeking from between her legs drinking a glass of water while the staff stood around waiting patiently for the next contraction.

After she finished drinking I told her, "*Hisa habibti, shidi bidun talec, aashan ma titmazaish*" which loosely translates to, "Now my dear, push without a contraction, so you won't tear." So she pushed, slowly and gently, and I protected the perineum as best I could, and the head came out; afterward the body followed, and whoops! I put the baby on her mother's belly.

But Demerol has unwanted side effects, and the baby was born a little flaccid, with low muscle tone and not really wanting to breathe, so we had to convince her to start breathing. Finally she was persuaded and started crying loudly, but not before we called a pediatrician, who did not come, which caused some tension and anger in those present; a really unnecessary addition to a lovely birth. But in the end, all was well and the baby was put in her mother's arms.

The baby's weight was 8 pounds, and the perineum was intact. I was really proud and still am, as if it was my own perineum. I'm proud not of the fact that it didn't tear, but that I did not give in to peer pressure and perform the cut, and also that I correctly evaluated the flexibility of the perineum, and saved her from unnecessary pain after birth. I know that in the coming months there will be many occasions when I will not be able to stand the pressure and that I will perform redundant episiotomies, so it was uplifting to experience such a success.

My supervisor, by the way, did not say a word about it but simply slipped away as it was already the end of her shift.

I was also present today at a C-section that was brought on because of a breech birth. The baby came out with a very strange head, without a lot of neck and with ears that hung a little too low on his head. And yet it was unclear whether this was because of his position in the uterus, or because of a syndrome.

Our hospital is located in an area where intermarriage is quite common, and thus we come across many congenital syndromes. These are often discovered only at birth, as the mothers do not follow up throughout the pregnancy regularly or thoroughly. I hope this time it will work out.

So this is the day's harvest, and we'll see what will tomorrow bring.

You first need to get their attention

I have a supervisor that constantly shouts. It's not even shouting, really... it's more like screaming. And whatever she screams about is so irrational that calm and logical answers or explanations do not really help. She screams at the nurses, the doctors, the hospital director and the head nun. The situation is so absurd that most of the time when she screams at people, no one, including me, gets worked up or offended. It's a bit like a situation in which a madman is screaming in the street - no one feels any anger toward him; only pity.

By the way, there is only one nurse who doesn't get screamed at by Miriam, and one day I asked her what her secret was. She smiled mysteriously and invited me to a cup of tea on the balcony, where she said in a heavy Russian accent:

"One day, fifteen years ago, when I first started working here, Miriam began to shout at me. I told her, 'Miriam, you do not shout at me.' She continued to shout and I said again, 'Do not shout at me,' and I hit my hand on the table so hard my wedding ring flew to the floor.

"Miriam started shouting again and I told her, 'If you continue to shout at me I'm going to take this chair and bash your head with it.' Miriam continued to shout so I raised my chair high in the air and then she stopped shouting and said, 'Vera, what's wrong with you? Are you crazy?' So I said, 'Yes! I'm crazy! And if you do not stop shouting, this chair is coming for your head.'"

I asked her why she wasn't fired and she smiled and replied that she did not know but since that day, Miriam hasn't screamed at her any more.

I don't have the courage to threaten her with a chair, which is probably the only thing that would work. Most of the time I'm fine with it but sometimes it's just too much. I arrive at work feeling joyless when I know that there might be a day of shouting and scolding ahead, even if it is nothing personal. Add to that the fact that I'm new and being scrutinized by everyone, and that due to the staff's many hidden wars, everyone gets criticized for everything from everyone all the time and one winds up with a general feeling that is extremely unpleasant.

I don't want to grow a thick skin; I want to work in a place where I feel safe just being myself and not having to stay on alert all the time, constantly defensive and thinking how to phrase each sentence so as not to step on anyone's toes - and there are thousands of these metaphorical toes scattered around like mines on a battlefield. This situation does not allow for fruitful learning, or fruitful anything for that matter. If I were a potted plant, I would wilt.

Here is an example: we had a case of shoulder dystocia this week. The woman was giving birth for the fifth time and the estimated weight of the baby was seven and a half pounds. She had given birth in the past to babies with a similar weight, never over eight and a half pounds. The delivery was moving along wonderfully, the head descended quickly and there was no reason to expect shoulder dystocia (as is usually the case, unfortunately). So of course I did not do an episiotomy. As it turns out, the baby's weight was eleven and a half pounds, and by the way, the woman wasn't even scratched.

Once the baby was born, after a lot of stress and the help of two midwives and two doctors who pressed on her belly from every possible direction, Miriam entered the room and screamed, "Why didn't you give her an episiotomy!!" She really let it rip. When she screamed, I couldn't get a word in edgeways, so later I tried to have a calm conversation with her about the matter, asking her why on earth should I have given the woman an episiotomy, how could I have predicted such an event, and why none of the experienced and well-educated staff who were also in the room with me, and there were several of those, had not even hinted about that course of action. My efforts were rewarded with a second dose of screaming.

Tomorrow I have a morning shift, on the busiest day of the week: C-section day. There are two planned, but they always manage to squeeze in two or three more. It's very dangerous to enter our delivery room on a Tuesday. It's likely you'll find yourself in the operating room.

I'm looking for a way out. This week I sent a resume to the hospital where I did my internship, even though I know they have no available positions. I'm crossing my fingers.

The story of how we saved a woman's life (after we almost killed her...)

Yesterday I had a crazy evening shift. Reception was full of women who were vomiting, fainting or about to give birth; the emergency room was full of women with abdominal pain, headaches or bleeding; we had three normal births and one vacuum delivery, two C-sections, a manual extraction of a placenta in one of the births and massive postpartum bleeding in another.

In addition, we had a woman with severe preeclampsia who was given magnesium, two women who had already undergone C-sections, and five women in various stages of premature labor, and all this with a staff of three midwives and a nurse. It was a great shift for learning how to work under pressure, how to be flexible, how to make split-second decisions, how to work accurately and efficiently, how to prioritize and so on. The midwives on the shift with me were wonderful, so all in all we worked really well and it felt good to work together, except during some stressful parts when I felt I wasn't truly able to handle everything at once.

So the story of the woman whose life we saved began quite well. It was her first birth, and she walked around with her husband in the reception room until she was 5 centimeters dilated and then went into the delivery room. The doctor broke her waters straight away and gave her a terrible stripping[37] - a recurring motif with all

---

37 Stripping, also called 'manual separation of the membranes' is a separation between the uterine wall and the amniotic sac during a vaginal examination

the women who gave birth yesterday. The delivery was progressing at a steady pace. She actually wanted an epidural, but the anesthesiologist was dealing with a C-section and by the time he arrived, she was fully dilated. The woman began to push and was doing well, as the baby slowly descended down into this world. Then the monitor began to show heartbeat decelerations, which in my opinion were not serious. In between contractions the pulse recovered nicely. All in all, these were variable decelerations that are common during this stage of labor.

But the doctor was stressed out (as he is all the time) and he told me, "Dismantle the bed and tell her to start pushing and I'll put pressure on her belly." Of course it was too early, even for pressing on the belly, so he decided to use the vacuum.

Well, we brought out the vacuum and called in another doctor to put pressure on the abdomen. Then Dr. Stressed Out gave her an episiotomy the size of the Gulf of Suez, the baby was born with an Apgar score of 9-10, and it all ended well.

Or maybe it did not end so well, because the woman started bleeding from the episiotomy. There was a scary amount of blood. Before the birth she had had a hemoglobin level of 12.6 and after the birth it went down to 8.5. That means she had lost about four units of blood. Within two minutes, she had a pulse of 150 and

---

using a finger. The action results in the release of prostaglandins from the cervix, causing contractions and the progress of labor. Stripping is usually quite painful and you need to obtain the consent of the woman before the procedure. Unfortunately I found that many cases of stripping are done without the consent of the woman and without any explanation, including one case that would be considered rape in every way. The woman screamed, "Stop, get your hand out, you're hurting me!!" and the doctor ignored her completely and continued to brutally dig into her vagina. It happened when I was still in my internship and although I filed a complaint against the doctor, nothing came of it. I think that the woman should have filed a police complaint.

blood pressure of 80/40; in other words she was in a state of shock. She turned pale and so did we. We almost killed her.

Afterwards, we saved her life. Within two minutes, we had taken blood tests, ordered two units of blood from the blood bank and given her another transfusion. The anesthesiologist began to revive her by giving her medication to stabilize her blood pressure, and she was given an oxygen mask. The anesthesiologist also put her to sleep so we could quickly stitch her terrifying episiotomy. The delivery room became an intensive care room, and well done us! We saved her! Hooray!

The woman and her husband thanked me afterwards and congratulated us on how well we'd treated her, and I wanted to bury myself in the ground out of shame. So when someone tells you how safe it is to give birth in a hospital, make sure to tell him about this case, and how hospitals are really good at untangling their own messes.

On the other hand, we had a C-section yesterday that really did save the life of the baby and his mother. It was a case of a serious placenta separation in week thirty-two. Without hospital treatment, this baby, and probably his mother too, would not be alive today.

Twenty-four hours straight in the delivery room

An evening shift; sleeping in the delivery room as backup - luckily no one woke me up - followed by a day shift. Both of these were filled to the brim with activities and stories that could make a nice script for some American soap opera. For example, there was the story of a woman who had already undergone four C-sections, in one of which the baby was stillborn. Now she had another stillborn baby at week thirty-five, and had her final C-section today. She agreed to a tubal ligation. Imagine going through a C-section twice without getting to hold your baby at the end of it. At home she has three daughters. The two babies who died were boys, and may have suffered some genetic disease that only affects males.

The woman and her husband were just lovely, gentle and affectionate. The woman wasn't sure whether to have a tubal ligation but the husband was actually the one who encouraged her to do so and told her, "We have three wonderful daughters in good health, why should we risk you and why should you suffer so again?" I mention this because usually the husbands we encounter are not willing to allow their wives to undergo tubal ligation, and certainly not if they have only daughters.

Another woman arrived in week forty-two; that is, two weeks after her expected delivery date. The pregnancy was the result of an *in vitro* fertilization, after six years of infertility. She was thirty-five years old and therefore, according to the doctors, she had to have a C-section. Here every woman over the age of thirty who has not previously given birth is considered "too old." "You can't give birth vaginally," they told her, "it is very dangerous for you, why should you?" I immediately thought about myself. I'm thirty-one - so what, I'll be "too old" as well?

The last story of the shift was the saddest. It was that of a young woman, twenty-three years old, who is the second wife in a bigamous marriage to a fifty-five-year-old man from one of the Arab villages. Yes, there is still such a thing in our time, here in Israel. It isn't legal, but it exists. The husband and his first wife have subjugated her and in fact use her as a slave in their house. Since she has no health insurance in Israel, as she is originally from Jordan, her husband wanted her to be admitted to the hospital only if she would give birth the same day, in order to lower the cost of hospitalization as much as possible. But when she arrived, it turned out that the baby was in a breech position and that she had to give birth by C-section. I could actually see the husband calculating how much all these days of hospitalization would cost him.

And the worst thing was that she gave birth to a girl. His first wife had borne him four sons. One of the nurses told me this woman's fate would be quite bad. When her husband dies she will probably be deported with her daughter, since the sons of his first wife come first in terms of inheritance and they would not want to share anything with the other, lesser, woman.

After the end of my shift, all kinds of thoughts were running through my head, thoughts about the lives of all these women, with their complications and troubles and joys. For example, I asked myself whose life was more difficult, that of the woman who experienced the death of an unborn child twice and who had had five C-sections, but who has a wonderful husband who loves her and cares about her; or the life of a woman who was sold as a slave to her significantly older and uncaring husband (to say the least) but who had a healthy baby. At one point, I felt it was just too much to process in two days, too many lives that require deep attention and I didn't have enough to give each what she needed.

In fact, each of these women should have had her own midwife, someone to acknowledge her and understand her and accompany her through all the stages of birth, without her having to meet and get to know a new team every time. I didn't even tell you about another three births I attended on that shift: one a difficult vacuum birth; another a C-section - a woman in week eighteen of her pregnancy with a stillborn baby that she had been trying to deliver for three days now; and a woman in early pregnancy with triplets, conceived after a fourth IVF attempt, with a threatened abortion.[38] How can one process all of this?

38 Threatened abortion – in about one third of pregnancies, the slight bleeding that appears during early pregnancy may indicate the beginning of a miscarriage. Most cases end with a healthy pregnancy, and only a fraction of the cases will end in a complete miscarriage.

"I want a natural birth!"

This was the first thing she said to me; a beautiful and well-dressed woman who had just come to reception. Speaking clearly and pleasantly, she told me that she had taken a prenatal course and that it was really important that I help her to give birth without pain medication, breastfeed after birth and have a different experience from the one she'd had during her first birth.

I wanted to whisper to her, "Then run away from here!" But instead I assured her that I love natural births and that I would try to help her as much as I could. To myself I added that it would be best if she gave birth during my shift. She was giving birth for the second time and had a dilation of 4 centimeters. Giving birth for the second time is often speedier, so there was a good chance that she would succeed in delivering during my shift. She asked for an enema and then walked around a bit before entering the delivery room. I decided to be bold and put her on a physiotherapy ball instead of on the bed, like an overturned tortoise. She sat on the ball, jumped up and down and moved her hips in slow circular motion and said, "It's great, it really helps!"

After two minutes of natural birth, Dr. Elias, the chief physician entered and said, "How wonderful, she's sitting on the ball!" For a moment I thought I was dreaming, but then he burst my bubble by saying, "Great, so now get on the bed and Dana will break your waters." I tried to squeak, "But the woman is interested in a completely natural birth," but he snapped back at me and said,

"Excellent, there is nothing more natural than the breaking of the waters![39]"

That concluded our time on the ball. In order to break someone's waters, I first have to put in an IV drip and the woman needs to lie down on the bed. After that, the hospital's protocols don't allow the woman to get out of bed.

After her waters broke, her contractions became much stronger (as expected) and the woman had a pretty hard time, but she was determined not to take any painkillers. I showed her how to

39 A few words about water breakage: About one fifth of births begin with the waters breaking spontaneously. Most women will begin to have contractions and give birth within a day of this happening. Different hospitals have different policies regarding when to propose labor induction in the case of a woman whose waters have broken, but who is not having contractions. Some hospitals offer induction immediately following the breaking of waters, and in some cases it is acceptable to wait even a few days. In case the birth does not progress, the woman will be advised to take antibiotics to prevent the development of infection in the uterus. The rest of births begin without the waters breaking and the amniotic sac may break at any stage of the delivery - at the beginning, at a more advanced stage, or, in rare cases, even after the delivery. One of the most common medical interventions in hospitals is the artificial rupture of membranes, which causes the waters to break. In some hospitals, this is a routine action performed in order to speed up the delivery, even without a medical necessity. Other reasons for artificial rupture of membranes may include the induction of labor when it is not advancing; the need to place an internal monitor on the top of the fetus' head or the need to perform intrauterine transfusion, when the volume of waters is low and there are serious FHR decelerations. When a delivery advances properly and FHR is normal, there is no reason to break the waters, since this action also increases the chances of complications such as intrauterine infection or umbilical cord prolapse into the vagina. When the waters break, whether proactively or spontaneously, often there is a sharp increase in the level of pain experienced by the woman, and often if the water breaks during an early stage of birth, the woman will need pain relief medication sooner.

breathe and massaged her lower back. Her husband gently played with her hair and whispered words of encouragement. We successfully endured all of the contractions until at some point the husband said, "Now she is 8 centimeters dilated." I checked her and indeed she was. After a while he told me, "Now she has a dilation of nine and a half," and again, she had. Then she gave birth, and in between her few last contractions, she said, "How lucky that I had a chance to give birth during your shift."

After the birth, she asked to breastfeed the baby, but the midwife who was with me claimed that the baby was breathing heavily (although the neonatal doctor didn't think so – we had called her because the amniotic fluid had meconium in it). Anyway, the baby went straight to the nursery.

The most annoying thing was that Dr. Elias asked me afterwards: "Well, did you break her waters?" When I replied in the affirmative, he said, "Well done, that's how I like it. I'm really pleased with your work and I am happy to see that we are likeminded." Ugh.

I told the head nurse that I felt really desperate and that I don't really see a future in this type of work. I'm preparing the ground for my departure.

Take a number and stand in line

This is what the chief nurse from the hospital where I had my internship said to me. They had no vacancies in the delivery room at the moment, but I should get on the list. So in a month I intend to leave the monastery (doesn't it sound exotic?) and go to work in the Pediatric Department at my beloved hospital until a position becomes available in the delivery room.

This is not an easy decision. On the one hand, I am currently working in a delivery room, cutting my teeth and gaining experience. Even if my approach is not compatible with that of the hospital, I am still learning. If I leave, I won't be able to work as a midwife for an unknown period of time. On the other hand, you know what kind of delivery room I'm working in. Yesterday, for example, I had a shift with three vacuum births, a C-section and one vaginal delivery with shoulder dystocia. There are a huge percentage of interventions during childbirth there.

I informed Miriam, my head nurse, in what was a very pleasant conversation considering the circumstances. She did not scream at me or try to emotionally blackmail me, something that would really have intimidated me. Tomorrow I meet with the hospital's chief nurse, so wish me luck!

I started to say goodbye to this strange hospital...

Goodbye to Dr. Stella, the melancholy doctor from the Czech Republic, who had studied in her native country and was now married to an Israeli-Arab physician. To this day, she regrets boarding the plane with him for Israel; she is always dreaming of going back home to her parents' farm, knowing nevertheless that she'll never leave her children here.

Goodbye to Dr. Karim, whom I once saw sitting on the floor and bursting into tears when he could not pull a baby out with the vacuum.

Goodbye to Dr. Elias, head of the delivery room; a man 6 ½ feet tall, who gives women no choice regarding how they want to have their birth.

Goodbye to Miriam, who still shouts at people and probably will never cease.

Goodbye to Hasna, the strange nursing assistant from Jordan; brown-skinned, shaped like a triangle, sixty years old, unmarried, who lives with her sister in the convent and busies herself with gossiping and cooking.

Goodbye to ward rounds with seven doctors peering together into the vagina of a helpless woman, with no respect and no privacy.

Goodbye to violent births.

Goodbye to lonely babies.

Goodbye to Sister Mona, the most diligent and frustrated nun in the world, about whom I still can't decide if she was a good friend or a gossiping schemer.

Goodbye to Sister Mary Paul, the kindest old nun in the whole world. Sorry I didn't understand a word you were saying.

Goodbye to wonderful food: spicy chicken and stuffed grape leaves, hummus with whole chickpeas for breakfast and a hot cinnamon and nut beverage for the new mothers.

Goodbye to all those women who gave birth here. I tried to help you but I'm not sure I could. I wish I had found the strength to stay.

I learned a lot, mostly about what I do not want in my life; and this is usually the most important lesson.

Getting one step closer

Nearly two weeks in the new hospital. I'm trying not to form any opinions on things too fast, so I've refrained from writing until now, so as not to set my mind in a certain direction. My opinion is still in the making, but yesterday I could say that I enjoyed my shift and that's something.

Everyone who knows the people involved advises me to take a deep breath and count to a thousand. Well, I took one and the truth is that it's not so bad. I can finally wear colored socks and not only white ones; Mother Superior isn't spying on me anymore. Also, the medical team is quite nice, although I have a feeling that not everyone can be trusted. Yesterday I came across an ugly example of someone telling tales on another nurse.

The ward's head nurse is a real character too. A classic case of someone who was appointed to be in charge of something dear to her, who became a bit of a tyrant, like a mother wolf protecting her cubs. She, too, is the shouting type, but as far as I've noticed, she never shouts without a reason. It's always when someone has made or is about to make a dangerous mistake, such as leaving an eight month old baby on an open high crib, or not preventing a child from trying to put something into an electrical outlet. Fortunately, she really loves me - probably from the days when I was there as a nursing student, and this works for me in the meantime. In truth, I'm beginning to like her. She is not a bad person, just very aggressive and uncompromising, which sometimes is perceived as meanness, and in my opinion unjustly so.

She is also highly professional, which is very refreshing. Her capabilities border on those of a soothsayer. She can, for example, diagnose the type of bacteria that lives in a wound according to its smell. The doctors, however, wait for the culture result and in the meantime treat the wound with the wrong type of antibiotics and it gets worse. After three days, the results come from the laboratory and confirm what she has said, and then they change the treatment. I swear I'm not making this up; it happened just this week to a child whose leg had been amputated and the stump got infected. She can smell an infant's diarrhea and know if it's dysentery or some other kind of germ. She looks at a child and by the color of his face diagnoses bowel intussusception in two seconds. What can you do? Thirty-five years of working with children does make a difference.

Besides, it is very important to her that nurses work as nurses and not as secretaries. To her, there is no such thing as a nurse who runs after a doctor the whole day reminding him of something he muttered during rounds. To her, everyone has to take responsibility for his or her part of the treatment and that's something I have dreamed of seeing since I finished nursing school. This frees the nurses to do what they're supposed to. Doctors, to her, are completely independent and do not need a nurse to hold their hand, as unfortunately happens in many other places. And if suddenly a doctor misbehaves to a patient or nurse, she screams at him and humiliates him before his supervisor...that's the less positive side of her, the one that has earned her the reputation of being a monster.

The Pediatrics Department. With all hospitalized children, I always wonder how many actually have to be here and how many would have been able to have the same care at home and get well. I still can't answer that question, but there are cases where there is no doubt that a child has to be hospitalized, such as the case of a child aged three-and-a-half, whose leg got amputated during an accident at his home. Explain to me who lets a child that age play with a forklift? Then there is the two-month-old baby girl who hasn't gained a single ounce since birth and is currently undergoing a comprehensive diagnosis; not to mention the child with severe asthma and the one with bacterial meningitis.

There are other cases, however, in which it is clear, at least to me, that the child shouldn't be in the hospital. For example, the three-month-old baby who had a fever of 99.6°F at night and was brought in for a comprehensive diagnosis that includes lumbar puncture, blood tests and urine cultures, which at this age involves extracting the urine with a syringe through the abdomen. All completely unnecessary in my opinion and, by the way, in the opinion of the other nurses here, who are much more experienced than I.

Where does the problem lie? In fear. Every once in a while, there is an article in the newspaper about a baby who came to the emergency room with a high fever, was released, and then died a few hours later from some violent bacteria. Rare and sad cases, and when they happen you can be sure that no child with a fever is going to be released from any emergency room in the next few months before going through every known test.

It also seems to me that much of the problem lies not in the system but in parents who do not want to know about or cannot handle a little fever, or half a day of diarrhea and vomiting. So they run straight away to the ER, hospitalize their child, and agree to every possible test and intravenous antibiotic therapy, sometimes including several types of antibiotics. In most cases, after two or three days of repeated negative culture results, it turns out that the fever was caused by a virus. The antibiotic is thus stopped and if the child hasn't contracted a real disease in the meantime, he can go home.

Then again, there are still those cases in which all of this hassle saves lives. And it is sometimes impossible to know which of the children who visit the emergency room today are the ones who should stay. This is not an ideal situation, and this is not an ideal world.

And then there are the parents, of course. So many parents make nurses out to be liars. They say to their child, "No, she did not come for you" (sure I did); or, "don't worry, she is not about to give you medication" (I certainly am); or, "She doesn't want to take your temperature" (really?); or, "This is over!" (What's over? We're just getting started) and so on.

No one tries to explain to the child, however big or small he is, about what they are going to do to him; if it will hurt or just be irritating, if a medicine has a bitter taste or how long the procedure will take. Why do they act this way? They are probably afraid that the truth will frighten the child. But I believe that lies are much more frightening, especially when the truth comes out ten seconds later. Maybe they are afraid that the child will not cooperate (it's his right, isn't it?) or that the child will get upset with them. They prefer him to be angry at the nurse.

In fact, I too would rather he be angry with me and not with his parents, but their lies do not really contribute to that. They expect me to play along with their lies, like, "You're not going to give him a shot, right?" or, "It will not hurt, right?" and that I will not do. I prefer to tell the truth. "I want to change your bandages. It might be unpleasant but it's not supposed to hurt. If it hurts, tell me and I'll try to do it more slowly."

And there is also the issue of, "Don't cry, be a good boy." Why wouldn't children cry, especially the little ones, say, a girl of eighteen months, who has yet to develop verbal skills. She doesn't even have the ability to resist her parents or me. Why wouldn't she cry and express her protest in the only way she can? Why teach children from a young age that *a good boy = a child who doesn't cry*? I actually tell parents, "It does not bother me that they cry, and maybe it helps them. A lot of adults also cry when they get such treatment."

Not all parents are like that, but unfortunately almost all the parents I encountered have been at least until now. I hope I'll meet others.

And one small yet important positive thing: in the ward, there is a general concept that one should not interrupt a child's sleep unless there is a really good reason. For example, they try not to dispense medication during the night, and do not take a child's temperature or bother him for no good reason. During the day as well, a sleeping child is rarely woken up. I like this very much and I think we need to act this way in all departments, not just pediatrics. Sleep is a great healer; antibiotics only help a little.

I finally managed to complete the practical part of my midwifery course.

I'm pregnant!

Somehow I never imagined it would happen to me. The wonder of it all still fills me from the inside.

"Oh my, am I really pregnant? Really and truly?" I still have parts of me that refuse to believe it, and I have difficulty understanding what it means. A guest is staying over at our house now, a friend from the Netherlands. Suddenly there's another person in the house. I thought about how in a few months a new person will join us, but this time it will not be for a week or two, but for many years more. It is very strange to think of it this way. Such a thing has never happened to us before, that someone came to visit and stayed forever.

I look at the reality of our lives as they are today and tell myself that it's about to change, drastically. So many unexpected surprises and changes await us, and something in me is happy about it, and something is fearful. There is a part of me that does not know if we can handle it, while another part knows that we can. These feelings must be familiar to women who have been pregnant.

There are also preparations and important decisions that should be made, or at least contemplated. For example, we do not know the gender of the fetus yet, but nevertheless, we have decided not to do a circumcision, in case it is a boy. We also decided that we will try to use reusable diapers, so I read a lot about those and my mother has already prepared about twenty of them (thanks, Mom!). There are lots of big and small decisions and all sorts of little details for which you can prepare. But I know full well that most things will remain a surprise and will reveal themselves over time.

Over the last two weeks, the question of where to give birth began to be raised. So far it was just something to reflect upon, but suddenly it became an important question to be seriously examined and for which a decision must be made. I'm not really that eager to give birth in a hospital, but I also know that if I have to, for some reason, it'll be fine. Of all the hospitals, I prefer my home turf of course, but I know that for me it would probably be less than optimal to give birth there, as the staff is sure to take an interest in my wellbeing and I probably will not have much privacy during my birth. This is how it was when I came to have a general review. I had an appointment with one doctor but in the end there were four doctors in the room, who just came to see that all was well.

But let us put the matter of hospitals to the side for now. How about giving birth at home? This is a great option but a bit tricky, because I live quite far from a hospital. It's a thirty-five minute drive, if you do not get stuck behind a truck. It's a bit risky, but doesn't necessarily rule the possibility out. I'm supposed to have a meeting with a homebirth midwife sometime soon and make a decision about it.

Other options that come to mind - and here we enter the realm of fantasy - are giving birth at a guesthouse near the hospital, and hoping that the birth won't happen on a weekend, otherwise the other guests will have an unforgettable experience; or, my favorite, giving birth at home by mistake.

Also, it is not clear to me who I want there. A part of me wants to be alone. Oh well, a midwife will be in the next room, but I don't want to be disturbed at all. Another part thinks about what fun it would be to get a lower back massage. I have no idea how I will cope with the pain or if I'll want someone beside me or not. But I have a feeling that these matters are becoming clearer inside me and will come to fruition sometime soon.

Another part of me has been speculating even more about what will happen after the birth. Things like breastfeeding, lifestyle changes, the baby growing up, us maturing as parents, about what kind of mother I am going to be and what kind of father Eitan will be. How our newborn will integrate into our community, and who his or her friends will be - there are some potential candidates; they too are currently embryos or tiny babies.

Wow, everything is about to change.

Having just re-read what I wrote, it seems to me that it gives an impression of confusion or agitation. But I do not feel that way at all. Instead, I feel rather peaceful and with a stable center of gravity. Things will become clear if I only give them time. And on the whole, it's kind of fun to ponder all these things, to fantasize a little, to think about baby names, to move my hand softly across my belly. I'm still working in the pediatrics department, but from next week I am going to cut down a bit on my hours. I'm also still doing a million other things, but little by little I am finding someone to take over my different tasks, taking on fewer responsibilities and making room for what is about to come.

And we weren't taught any of this during our midwifery course.

It is time for us to talk about how our Ya'ara was born.

It happened just a month ago; the problem is that whenever I try to sit down and write, she wakes up and cries. I think that babies have a high sensitivity to situations in which we, the parents, are just enjoying ourselves, and so they wake up.

The original plan was to give birth in a birth center in the garden of a midwife who lives close to a hospital. We met her several times and it looked promising. However, a small inner voice kept telling me, "This will not happen."

I felt great and had a healthy pregnancy until week thirty-six, when my blood pressure started to rise and, at the end of week thirty-seven, I checked myself into the maternity ward at the hospital where I work, after my gynecologist refused to see me or let me have blood and urine tests as part of my HMO coverage. I wanted to find out if I had toxemia (preeclampsia[40]). During my hospital-

---

40 A few words about preeclampsia: five percent of all pregnancies show symptoms of preeclampsia, which is triggered by unknown factors. Preeclampsia is characterized by high blood pressure, which appears after week twenty of the pregnancy, and the appearance of proteinuria and edemas. In more severe cases, there may be damage to other organs such as the liver, kidney and brain, and in very rare cases it might cause death. The placenta may also be affected, and as a result there might be interference with the growth of the fetus, a low level of amniotic fluid and placenta separation. In most cases, preeclampsia appears only towards the end of pregnancy and is very mild. In more complex cases, preeclampsia occurs relatively early and there is a dilemma over whether to terminate the pregnancy and have the risk of

ization it became clear that I had only slight preeclampsia, but it was not something you'd want to give birth at home with or while swimming with dolphins. And here began my real lesson, or maybe I need to think of it as my hands-on experience.

Before that, I had never been hospitalized, not even for a day. And now, here I was in a maternity ward: waiting, being monitored, and all the time discovering what it feels like to be hospitalized, having to take a shower in the hospital, eat hospital food, wait for the doctors' rounds and so on...

Obviously, my situation was still different from that of other patients, as this is my home turf, where I feel at home and know all the staff, from the midwives, nurses and doctors, to the X-ray technicians, porters, guards and department secretary. And yet, it was an interesting and eye-opening experience.

Perhaps the most important lesson I learned was about being flexible – not to expect to give birth exactly how I wanted, but rather to stress the important ingredients that needed to be present. And how to try and be at peace with each and every moment of this changing situation, which kept on changing during and after childbirth; how to make decisions based on what I was facing at the moment and not what I had wanted or imagined – not to say fantasized - back at home.

---

premature birth or to continue the pregnancy and risk the mother's wellbeing. There is no cure for preeclampsia except to give birth. Within a few days of birth the woman is out of danger. However, severe cases of preeclampsia are usually treated with a substance called magnesium sulfate that prevents the seizures that come as a result of the brain injury that preeclampsia may cause. Also, cases of high blood pressure can be treated with hypertension drugs. A significant part of prenatal care is designed to detect signs of preeclampsia (blood pressure measurements and taking urine samples) and every time a doctor or a nurse examines a pregnant woman they should ask her if she suffers from headaches, stomachaches or blurred vision, which can be a sign of the development of preeclampsia.

I think I was able to apply this lesson quite well, and I felt good almost all the time; very relaxed, with a lot of tranquility. There was also something good in this, the almost total detachment from domestic chores like laundry, walking the dog, working on the computer, meeting friends, etc. As time went by, I felt how I was reverting into myself, and it felt good to be on this island of tranquility.

I had a private room, painted blue and decorated with flowers and pictures my friends had brought me at the wonderful baby shower they organized, during which I got a massage from eight hands, a lot of reassurance and small joyful gifts. On the shelf was a small library of the books they had brought me to read. On the wall hung my personal shield, a special drawing I made while I was pregnant, which included drawings of elements I find strengthening and encouraging. So, in the week before my birth that was the little nest where I stayed most of the time. And what did I do?

Aside from reading, listening to music and sleeping, there were also attempts to start the labor. The reason was the preeclampsia, which was indeed mild, but preeclampsia by its nature never improves. It could have worsened or stayed as it was, and I was afraid of the most severe case, for which I would have had to take magnesium. The problem with taking magnesium is that I would not have been able to be with my baby for a day after the birth.[41] Besides, there were still two weeks until the estimated date of birth, which could easily turn into a month. And if I would have preeclampsia during this month I would need to be monitored, which the HMO said they would not do as an out-patient, so I'd have had to stay in the hospital anyway. And on top of that, the volume of amniotic

41 Magnesium is a drug given intravenously. Whilst being administered, the woman must be monitored closely in the delivery room – usually without her baby beside her, as he also needs to be monitored, due to the magnesium he was exposed to while still in the womb.

fluid was decreasing, which indicates a decline in the functioning of the placenta, which supplies all the needs of the fetus. This is another outcome of preeclampsia. I reached a severe decrease in amniotic fluid close to the end of my pregnancy.

But other than that, everything was fine. I felt good and the little life inside me felt good as well. Since my uterus probably wasn't about to give birth yet, we had to try and use everything we had in order to induce labor, and that meant prostaglandins deposits (I received five of them!), Prepidil gel, an Atad catheter and oxytocin.[42]

I got into a daily routine of waking up in the morning, taking a shower, having breakfast, going down to the delivery room, hooking myself up to a monitor, unhooking myself and getting a doctor to sign off on the procedure, and then discussing with him what we should do that day. We would decide together and then act accordingly. The one doctor who told me, "And then I'll decide what you should do" was chewed out badly by me.

Towards the afternoon, I would have contractions that lasted usually until one in the morning, and then they would die out and I would go to bed. The next day it was the same thing all over again, like a kind of a weird daytime entertainment.

---

42 These are all methods to induce labor. Prostaglandins: natural substances secreted in the cervix, which soften it and cause contractions. One method of induction includes the introduction of vaginal prostaglandins to ripen the cervix and cause a small opening to allow continued induction using Pitocin through transfusion. This induction method may cause strong contractions and therefore is not used with women who have previously undergone a C-section for fear of uterine rupture. Prepidil gel also belongs to the family of prostaglandins, but appears as a gel rather than as a suppository. Atad Catheter: two balloons inflated with water inserted into the cervix, which create a mechanical opening of the cervix. After twelve hours, the catheter is removed and induction begins via intravenous Pitocin drip, which is actually a synthetic oxytocin. The use of a catheter is suitable for women who have had a C-section in the past or women who do not react to prostaglandins (like me).

All this lasted one week. The eighth day began in the same way, and in the afternoon I started having painful contractions with short intervals between them. When it seemed that they might be a little different and a bit more powerful than they had been so far, I called one of the two friends who were going to be with me during my birth. The friend came, and along with Eitan, who had been there since morning, we passed those first few hours together. I mostly bounced on the physiotherapy ball, which made us laugh hysterically because my room overlooked the street, and when I jumped on the ball my head appeared and disappeared in the window, came and went, and somehow we found that very funny. My dear friend also helped a lot with massages, and the shower next to my room worked overtime that day. It soon became clear that it must be serious this time, and yet I did not want to go down to the delivery room. I knew it was too early.

So in this way we passed the time until ten in the evening - time flies when you're having fun... Every minute I had a contraction, and every contraction lasted about a minute. It was very painful, but mostly it was exhausting. Finally we went to the delivery room, because the nurses on the maternity ward were on to me – I guess the sounds I made were a bit disturbing.

In the delivery room, we received a warm welcome. After all, I had been coming and going for a week now without giving birth. I asked the midwife to check me. I had a dilation of one-and-a-half centimeters, which was actually a significant advance after a whole week without any progress, but still disappointing after hours of frequent contractions. It was then that I realized why midwives aren't really impressed by contractions caused by prostaglandin deposits. These contractions are very strong and close together, but not necessarily effective in terms of shortening the cervix and increasing dilation. Well, we made ourselves comfortable in the back room, which was pink and had a rope hanging from the ceiling. We positioned the blue physiotherapy ball, the CDs we had brought, and, of course, we hung my personal shield on the wall.

The contractions continued to come every minute at a constant pace, and grew in strength with each one. My other friend had arrived by now, and the massages the two of them gave me were just wonderful and actually helped me endure each contraction. All the while I inhaled, exhaled, made strange low sounds, and in general was very happy to know that it was probably going to happen that day!

But I also knew that it might take a while, because this was not a spontaneous labor, but an induced one. In general, it was interesting to see how on the one hand I was the patient now, but on the other I had not completely turned off the midwife within me. I followed the frequency of my contractions and checked the monitor to make sure that the FHR was okay, so I could quickly unhook myself from the machine. Only one thing I "forgot" and that was to ask the midwife to check my blood pressure. I was really afraid that it was very high, because of the pain of the contractions, and that I would have to be given magnesium.

Two lovely midwives arrived when the night shift started at 11 PM. They were Michal, who had been my instructor during my internship, and Olivia. I was hoping all the time that Michal would the one to attend my birth. She was not supposed to be at work at all, but someone else was sick and so they called her in unexpectedly. We greeted each other and hugged, and then she went to deliver other women who were actually about to give birth and not just pretending to be, like me, and left us to jump on the ball and moan.

After another hour, I went back to take a shower and a bath. The pain was just unbearable, the contractions were longer, and the breaks between them were almost gone. Michal came and asked if I wanted to be examined. On the one hand I knew that progress would encourage me, but on the other hand I knew that lack of progress would depress me. So we waited some more and at 1 AM I asked her to examine me. The dilation was one and a half centimeters, which meant there had been no change despite these intense few hours. It was very, very, very discouraging, and I didn't know how I was going to endure the hours ahead. I decided, along with Michal, to take an epidural. It seemed that I was going to have to personally undergo every existing procedure, myself.

I did not know how I would stay calm and not move when the epidural was being administered, because at that point the contractions were so strong that I had to shake myself in all directions. But Michal said I mustn't move and that I could make it, and so it was. The anesthesiologist was gentle and quick, so I really had only one contraction during which I couldn't move. Then came the wonderful calmness and rest and it didn't hurt anymore, and that was just a blessing. I sent my lovely companions to sleep in shifts in the maternity ward suite, and I tried to rest a little myself, because I knew there was a long road ahead of me yet.

After resting for about an hour, I decided that I had indulged myself enough and started inducing my own labor again. I stood on all fours, shook my hips, and even got off the bed and stood up which was possible despite the epidural. I wanted to allow gravity to do its work. Occasionally I also rested, because after all, I hadn't slept for almost a day.

In this fashion, I slowly advanced and when the shifts changed at seven in the morning, I was 4 centimeters dilated! And now we also had Nili with us, the beloved midwife who was in charge of the delivery room and who stayed until the end. Since that day was Purim, [43] Nili was dressed up as Minnie Mouse. It was so hilarious

43 Purim is a Jewish holiday, in which customs include giving charity to the poor, dressing up in costumes and being merry.

and surprising to see her mouse ears, nose and whiskers every time she entered the room. So now we had entered the morning shift, during which things ran smoothly. The epidural did its work, the contractions continued, and when the PG stopped having an effect they added Pitocin. Apparently I had to try that too. I rested and changed positions every once in a while, and it was pretty fun. At one point, a doctor suggested hooking up an IUP machine, which monitors contractions in the womb, but I told him that while it was very interesting for me to try everything, I did not really have to try *everything*.

Before noon, my dilation was 9 centimeters, and we were very happy. Nili even opened up the delivery kit, but at the same time she diagnosed an occipital posterior position. Oops. That's not so good. There are quite a lot of cases of deliveries that end in a C-section because of it. But there was nothing to do but continue to stand on all fours, move my pelvis, make sure that when I turned over in bed I did it from the correct side and through the abdomen, and hope that the fetus would turn around in there.

At this point, the epidural wore off and they asked me if I wanted more. I decided not to have another, because we were right at the end (yeah, right) and I wanted to feel when I entered the second stage of birth. I began to feel the contractions, which were weak at the beginning, but soon their power grew to the frightening intensity they had been before the epidural, and at the same wearying pace of one a minute, with no time to rest in between. It is funny that during the birth preparation courses I've given, I have always emphasized that there is a calm between each contraction and that even if it really, really hurts, you can always have a bit of rest in between... So apparently this is not always true.

My dilation remained at 9 centimeters for about the next two hours or so, until finally I begged for, and received, another epidural. At some point I was already fully dilated, the head was low and I began to feel pressure, as well as the contractions again.

A contraction every minute, every minute, every minute... I checked myself, and felt her head for the first time! Her head was soft and pleasant, so I started to believe that surely there was a baby in there and that this whole thing was actually happening. The pressure at this point was very strong and shook me with each contraction. I pushed standing up, on all fours, on the birth chair, leaning on my side, leaning on my back; I was basically short of standing on my head from trying everything, but the baby's head did not descend and didn't move even one millimeter.

It was a bit strange - Nili was busy with another birth at this point, so I acted as my own midwife, pushing, screaming, and then checking, showing no progress, and pushing again...

After another two hours like this, the pain was unbearable, and I was desperate. Nili entered and confirmed that there was no progress. At this point I began to cry like a little child. I cried about everything: about the pain, the pushing, the week in hospital trying to do everything to avoid surgery because of the preeclampsia and now it seemed that this was what would happen. I cried from frustration and despair and fear. The midwife in me, the one I could not seem to switch off, looked at what was happening with interest and commented, "Oh great, now she cries. Maybe something will finally move in there that way."

At this point I had another epidural, and Nili asked me to take a little rest and stop pushing, and to just let the contractions do their job. I lay on my side and waited and waited for the hospital's standard three hours for giving birth after reaching full-dilation to be over, so additional measures could be considered. After those three hours had passed, the physician who was to deliver Ya'ara, Dr. Solomon, came in and we decided to try to pull the baby out with vacuum, and if that failed, we would go to surgery. To carry out the vacuum we moved to the operating room, and the medical staff was asked to prepare the room just in case, so I also had the chance to experience the preparations for a C- section. The staff was so wonderful and gentle. Everything was done quietly; the anesthesiologist was supportive and gentle and wished me luck in such a cheerful way.

Strange, but it was at that point that I felt no fear; I was relaxed and felt that I was surrounded by love and support. Nili stayed with me, even though her shift had ended three hours ago, and the midwives of the new shift came in and encouraged me. Dr. Solomon was so serious and quiet, although usually he was such a clown.

Well, we reached the end of my journey. The doctor pulled, the doctor made a cut (what, I should have missed the opportunity to experience an episiotomy?) And I pushed, and within two or three contractions Ya'ara was lying on my belly. That's also when we found out that the baby was a girl. The pediatrician examined her and, although she had trouble breathing at first, it was quickly dealt with, and within two minutes she was given back to me. She had the most amazing look in her eyes and the most charming cry, which we now know is one of her unique characteristics; it goes like this: "Lhahaha, lhahaha, lhahaha."

So that was that. The birth was over, and looking back, I do not regret any part of it. And despite the fact that it was long and very painful, it didn't register as a traumatic or a negative experience. When I was in the recovery room, I started thinking about my next birth. What made the difference for me was the tremendous support I had received, from Eitan and my two friends, as well as from the wonderful staff of the delivery room. Another thing that made the difference was the fact that I'd had a say in all the decisions and never felt helpless at any stage.

So I completed this part of my education, and now I can truly be a midwife. I'm curious to see how my delivery will affect the midwife within me; my opinion towards interventions, vacuum births, epidurals and pain. I'm sure there will be an impact, but I'll have to wait and see what that will be. And when will I be back in the delivery room to find all that out? I do not know. But I'm planning to have a comeback soon.

Wishes do come true

In a month, I'll go back to working part-time in the delivery room of my beloved hospital! In the end, all my dreams have come true, and much earlier than I expected. On the one hand, it makes me very happy as I have been waiting for the moment when I will return to work; on the other hand, with every passing day, I think how can I part from Ya'ara for so many hours? If she sleeps for more than an hour, I already begin to miss her.

And what will it be like for her to be without me? She will mostly be with her father and for some time with a nanny. Who will breastfeed her? She will be six months old by then, but still, I feel apprehensive about it. But that's what's going to happen. Also, financially speaking, I have to go back to work, and the position is only part-time after all - only three shifts a week.

Right now she is sleeping on the living room carpet, all sweet and lovely. I love her. I did not know how much you can love another person.

I did not know that's actually what you get when you have a baby: love.

Comeback

For three weeks now I've been there, in the delivery room of my dreams, though until now my work has been limited to the reception desk. The entrance to the delivery room is through reception (except for those who have already given birth in the car…) and the general approach is that this is the place to start my orientation. This is how one gets familiarized with all the paperwork and programs on the computer, all the protocols and procedures. You would not believe how many forms there are to fill, how many labels there are to stick and how much typing needs to be done to admit a single woman. So here I am, and from the second day or so of my orientation I've been on my own most of the time, trying to manage all the new-yet-familiar details I have been bombarded with and to struggle with questions like, "Who to take care of first?" and, "Is it possible to find a way to pass up a vaginal examination?" and, "Where the hell is the ultrasound referral form?"

At least a quarter of my energy is being wasted on bureaucracy. Another quarter is wasted on finding doctors to come and sign admission or discharge forms. Another quarter goes into general disorientation... and everything is very confusing and stressful. The other day, for example, I sat quietly with a woman in reception, totally engaged in the form of occupational therapy called *preparing a hospital admission form*, when suddenly five women came to reception at once: two from the door, one from the window, one jumped out of the sink and another out of the computer (well, that's how it seemed, at least). Two of them were having premature contractions at week twenty-seven, one had just come for a routine check-up, one had fainted, and the last one… I can't remember.

And in the midst of all this mess I tried to be a hero and not run and ask the other midwives for help, even though I wanted to scream, "Help!" So I reassured myself, saying, "Calm down. Relax. Give this woman a urine sample cup and in the meantime sit the other two outside, connect the fourth one to a monitor and when the first one comes out of the bathroom, then you will..."

I try not to lose my head in all this, working out the right order of priorities, and after three weeks there I finally feel like I'm getting the hang of it and managing to get the job done. It's quite fun actually, like being able to juggle a lot of balls in the air at the same time.

One thing I would have loved to skip is the need to examine women at reception. Vaginal examination is not pleasant. In fact, I think it's safe to say that it's highly unpleasant, to say the least, and for some women the exam is very painful, frightening, scary... you name it. The cervix is often closed and it is very difficult to perform the test. It is important to explain to women that they can also refuse the test if there is no real need for it. Why, for example, should a woman who has been referred to us because of laryngitis in week twenty-five undergo a vaginal examination?

So, to sum all this up, here are two short stories from today. I was supposed to be in reception, but the first woman who came, told me in Arabic: "You're the midwife who delivered my Muhammad!" She was referring to the birth of her last child, while I was still in training. "But you gained weight," she added tactfully.

She asked for me to be her midwife this time too and my supervising midwife agreed to the arrangement. She had a wonderful birth. I showed her a way of breathing that helped her cope with the contractions and she practiced it all the way until the end. Finally, a cute baby was born, who looked just like his brother Muhammad, and all and all, it was really fun to deliver a woman whom I had delivered already. During the delivery I recalled all the details of her previous birth, and we exchanged experiences and memories.

Once her birth was over, I quickly drew some milk for Ya'ara and between breast A and breast B I was called in to the other delivery room to attend the delivery of a special woman, an Ethiopian who did not know a word of Hebrew except *yes* and *all right*. She also did not show when she was in pain, except for a very slight change in the wrinkles of her forehead and her respiratory rate. You had to be a real Sherlock Holmes to figure out that she was actually pushing. When the head was almost out, the midwife who was with me said, "This woman has given birth three times in Ethiopia, and none of them were in a hospital. She knows how to give birth. She doesn't need us, not really. So what do you say we put our gloves on but just look and not do anything?" Now you see why I love this delivery room?

So that's what we did, and she really didn't need us. The head came out, turned around, and the body followed. Gently and without shouting "Push, push" as she didn't understand Hebrew anyway, the baby came out. We didn't put our hands anywhere or protect the perineum, which didn't tear of course, and soon after, we put the baby onto its mother's chest, where, with great skill, she showed him the way to her dark nipple; how nice was that?

I spoke about this with Eitan, who replied in wonder, "So what are they paying you for, if you just sat there and did nothing?"

Whoever comes to the shift first wins a free delivery!

I already told you that many births take place during the shift changes in the hospital, which is why if you arrive a bit early there's a chance that a tired midwife from the previous shift will ask the fresh new midwife who just arrived to attend the birth. Yesterday morning I was the first to arrive for my shift. I heard the shouts of a late-stage delivery and peered inside a delivery room that was almost completely dark. A midwife greeted me with, "Dana! What are you looking at? Hurry up. Take a pair of gloves and you can receive this delivery!" So I put on some gloves, said hello to the woman and husband, got myself ready for the delivery, and during the next contraction she gave birth. The shortest delivery I've ever attended.

It turns out that the woman had arrived ten minutes earlier, fully dilated, and they didn't even have time to connect her to the monitor. The baby was tiny but very alert and alive, and brought much joy to his parents, who really wanted a son after three daughters.

By the way, most of the time it's not exactly correct to say that midwives want to leave immediately after each shift. Many of them will stay with the woman for an hour or even more to accompany her delivery until the end. The alternative, to be with a woman, develop with her a relationship of trust and endearment, become a part of her birth, and then leave just before the end, is very difficult - both for the mother and the midwife. If a midwife has to leave before the birth, she will usually call a few hours later to ask how the birth was, and of course she will come to visit the woman the next day on the maternity ward.

There is also a dark side to this. Sometimes such a strong relationship forms between the mother and the midwife that her replacement has a hard time stepping into the role of her predecessor, and the delivery ends with much less love and intimacy. I think a midwife who is about to leave should consciously prepare the ground for her coming departure, opening the way for the next midwife and slowly moving away from the mother to avoid a state of dependency. You can imagine how annoying it is to take care of a woman while her husband and mother keep saying, "The previous midwife was just lovely," and then adding with embarrassment when they notice my presence, "You're all lovely here of course!"

After this fun birth it was pretty quiet and we only monitored a few women from the maternity ward. A woman I had delivered two days earlier came to visit me before her release from the hospital and brought me some chocolates, olive oil and fragrant homemade olives. We kissed each other on both cheeks and I received an invitation to visit them in their village.

A delivery in the twenty-first century

The baby's heartbeat beeps in the background from the modern monitor.

We can tell how painful the contraction is by the intensity of the line displayed on the screen.

For pain, there's an epidural.

Blood pressure is measured automatically every thirty minutes.

The IV drips at a constant rate.

The birth is photographed and documented, by digital camera and video; the husband is already preparing a presentation of birth photos on his laptop.

When it gets too hot, we turn on the air conditioner.

The adjustable bed moves in every imaginable angle, without any need to get off of it.

After the baby is born, instant messages transmit the news to phones all over the country, with pictures, of course.

The umbilical blood is kept in a bag and from there it goes straight to the blood bank.

Sometimes I look at this whole situation from the side and am just amazed. How has our culture managed to take a completely natural process and overburden it?

And despite it all:

The man touches his wife; cheering, hugging and caressing.

The woman's body knows what to do, and she progresses with simplicity and speed.

A little poop still comes out during the last few contractions.

The woman is excited and tears up when the baby is born.

The father wants to cut the umbilical cord and is deeply moved by the process.

The baby is born with a wise and alert look in his eyes, searching for a nipple and wanting to be fed.

Some things never change.

Three women giving birth; three completely separate universes

One is giving birth for the first time, after her waters broke and without a lot of contractions, who has been in the delivery room since dusk, receiving induction but refusing painkillers, stuck for hours with a 4- centimeter dilation.

Another is giving birth for the fourth time, expecting a big baby and receiving induction because of it; stuck for hours with a head that won't descend into the birth canal.

The third is also giving birth for the first time, with normal contractions and an epidural.

One is secular, one a ultra-orthodox Jew, one an Arab woman from the village next to my house.

One has a smiling husband, another a nervous one, and the third has two friends.

Each progresses at a different pace; each room has a different atmosphere; each woman wants something different for her birth.

We were three midwives, each taking care of one woman; separate worlds that are not connected in any way, except that all of them contain women and that all of those women are giving birth.

Suddenly, the good fairy godmother of births came to the delivery room and with her silver wings touched the bellies of the three mothers. Within ten minutes all three gave birth. Three daughters came into the world. Three separate worlds that touched for a moment, and continued on their way.

It's part of life

On a scale of empty-quiet-calm-active-full-overwhelming, it was an active shift. This means that we worked constantly, and there were some peak moments of pressure, but we managed to find time to go to the bathroom, and even eat dinner together.

I tasked myself with assisting a woman who had arrived the day before and it just so happened that it had been me she met at reception. She came in with a doctor's reference sheet that read, "A routine ultrasound test, no pulse was observed in the fetus." This was in week thirty-two of her fourth pregnancy. She did not understand what it meant, because she was an immigrant from Ethiopia who had immigrated only a month ago and she didn't speak Hebrew. Fortunately there was an interpreter with her and we could explain the situation.

But it was so strange. She wasn't sad, at least not on the outside. She realized what was going on, nodded and smiled. At first I thought she was just introverted and reserved, as is the case with many Ethiopian women, but after yesterday I'm not sure that's the reason. But we'll get to that.

Immediately upon admission, the process of induction began. Beyond the emotional difficulty of continuing to be pregnant with a deceased fetus, it is a condition that can endanger the life of the woman as the fetus and the placenta begin to secrete substances into the mother's body, and within days or weeks can cause serious complications.

Yesterday a balloon had been placed in her cervix to induce labor, and when we arrived to our shift, she was already 3 centimeters dilated and receiving Pitocin. I volunteered to be with her and soon found myself facing a daunting stack of forms, which is always the case with a stillbirth, all of which had to be filled out and some of which had to be signed, and the woman, as I said, did not speak Hebrew.

She was alone. Her husband had gone to take care of their girls at home and none of the guides from the immigrant absorption center could stay with her, so it was only her and me and a pile of forms, and a nice telephone interpreter to help us. And so we communicated, in sign language and the language of the heart, and with one word I know in Amharic - *shint* - which means *to pee*, a very useful word during birth. Actually, I also know how to say *pharmacy* but I didn't find a way to slip it into the conversation.

At some point it seemed to me that something had changed. I mean, I say *seemed* because she couldn't tell me anything and because Ethiopian women are often so reserved that it's difficult to say when they are in pain. I explained to her, with my hands, that I wanted to examine her and she agreed. She was 5 centimeters dilated. We called the interpreter again and I asked her to explain to the woman all kind of things that would happen after the birth; and the woman had some questions too, such as would she be able to see the baby after birth and such. And that's it, we were alone again.

It was such a silent birth. Stillbirths are called that because the FHR does not make that rhythmic galloping horse's sound that you can hear on the monitor. But on top of that silence, was also the soundlessness of her being alone, of her not being able to verbally communicate with anyone, and her restraint in coping with the pain; a thick and heavy silence. I spoke to her and encouraged her, even though I knew she did not understand. I even hugged her and squeezed her hand and caressed her back, and smiled, and still she was quiet.

About an hour later, she suddenly started squatting on the bed and I heard a faint sound of her pushing. Then she moved one of her legs a bit and I realized she was actually giving birth. I could not tell her to "push" or "not to push," so I just put on gloves, and along with another midwife, who joined us at that point, just watched her giving birth; how you should truly give birth; how all of us should probably be giving birth. It was really amazing. The baby came out easily, and I cut the umbilical cord, which incidentally was bound tightly around the baby's neck. Maybe this was the reason for her death, but then again, maybe not.[44]Then the woman sat down, completely silent. She didn't think she was supposed to drop back onto the bed and lay down, exhausted, as most women do. She just sat cross-legged, ready for what was to come.

I wrapped the baby so she would look as nice as possible and showed it to her. She looked at her with interest and touched her head, looking for something. Then she looked at me in acknowledgement, and I took her away. The placenta came out easily and no stitches were needed. I thought she would want to lie down now, but she kept sitting on the bed, and when we helped her move to a clean bed, she still just sat there. Then I brought some water to wash her. You have to understand, all the women I have

---

44 A few words on the umbilical cord getting wrapped around the neck: a lot of people are horrified when they hear - or worse, when they see - a baby born with an umbilical cord around the neck. They are sure that the baby was in danger or perhaps suffered some serious injury. In fact, in a quarter of births, the umbilical cord is wrapped around the baby's neck, and sometimes around the body, arm or leg. In most cases, this has no meaning and it is revealed only after the birth. Sometimes it causes decelerations in the baby's pulse, which too are mostly meaningless. Sometimes the umbilical cord is wrapped several times around the neck (the most I've seen was four times). This can cause severe decelerations in FHR during labor but may also result in... nothing. You cannot predict its effect, so there is no significance to the discovery of this phenomenon in a prenatal ultrasound. When the baby is born, the midwife untangles the cord from around the neck, sometimes even at the moment that the head was born and the body still inside. There is no need for any follow-up or special tests after the delivery.

delivered to date have enjoyed the warm water that washes over them as they lie, but I've never seen a woman participating in the washing process. This woman began to wash herself, and it seemed so natural that I suddenly felt strange that other women do not do it as well. Then she washed her hands, face and mouth and drank a cup of hot sweet tea with cake.

I looked at her in surprise, full of questions. I wanted to ask her how she felt and what was going on inside her; was she sad or relieved? Has this happened to her before in Ethiopia? But due to the language barrier I would not have received any response to my inquiries and so I could only look at her and try to sense what she felt. What I felt from her was something like this:

"I feel very good right now, because the birth is over. I knew I would have a stillbirth, but it is something that happens to many women. Many women also lose babies that were born alive and a lot of women also die during pregnancy or childbirth. It's sad but it's just part of life and nature and I accept that and am glad I am healthy now and can go back to my daughters and my husband who are waiting for me at home. Everything that happens here now is a little strange to me because I gave birth to my daughters in a hut in Ethiopia and the experience was very different. I'm glad I met only women during birth and that there were no men there. I only wish my mother was here now and that I could sleep in my own bed tonight."

I cannot explain it. Although the situation was really sad, I could not feel sadness around this woman. I just felt how completely natural it all was. That is what I picked up in the air around her: complete acceptance, no anger and no self-pity, and a great ability to be herself, to be with her body, to give birth and move on.

Nobody gets out of bed in the middle of the night for no good reason

I mean that during the night shift, usually only the really urgent cases arrive. All the women with false labor contractions usually wait until morning or until their husbands come back from work. When we got to the shift the delivery room was completely empty, so while drinking coffee and eating cookies - a sure recipe for nausea at night - we planned who would to go to sleep and when. Then I pumped some milk in front of the on-duty doctor (he'd seen more intimate parts of me) and we chatted a bit. Suddenly, we saw a car screech to a halt and a man jumped out and yelled:

"Come quickly, my wife is giving birth in the car!"

I ran outside with a wheelchair and meanwhile another midwife opened a birth kit. It was the woman's fourth birth and she was 6 centimeters dilated. We quickly asked the important questions, such as "Do you have any allergies to medications" and "In what week of pregnancy are you?" and I put all the labels on all the forms and the other midwife put on gloves and in fifteen minutes the baby was out. It was very strange to see a woman just fifteen minutes before she gives birth. When you accompany her from the start you get acquainted, and then the pain gradually increases, and at the end, when she is all fired up and screaming, it seems like a natural extension of what happened before. But here we were introduced to a storm of a woman who was spewing fire and brimstone all around, shouting and waving her arms, throwing her head back and forth. It was just overwhelming.

At some point, I started talking to her in Arabic, because I thought that she would feel more comfortable if I'll talk in her mother tongue, and she looked at me with weird look and said in Hebrew to her husband, "I don't understand what she's saying." Probably my Arabic has a strange accent or something. And after she gave birth, what a surprise, another kind of person was revealed. Her whole face changed from a shrieking red to a calm pink full of sweetness and tenderness. She really glowed with her baby, how beautiful.

After this birth, I napped for about an hour, and when I awoke I made another cup of coffee and pumped some more milk in front of our transparent front door. It was real quiet, the only sound coming from the rain that kept pouring outside. Yael, the other midwife, was dozing a bit on a big armchair, when suddenly a car pulled to a screeching halt and a man jumped out and yelled:

"Come quickly, my wife is giving birth in the car!"

I ran outside with a wheelchair and this time we met a woman who was giving birth for the second time, with full dilation. Strangely enough, she came from the same village as the previous woman. She too was a screaming and flapping firestorm, all red and wild. Within five minutes she gave birth and, as if by magic, became a completely different woman a moment later.

It was quiet again until five in the morning, when another car screeched to a halt and a man jumped out and... I don't think I have to write the rest of the story, right?

This woman, who also came from the same village, had a really "slow" birth – she didn't' deliver until an hour after her arrival.

Probably someone had sprinkled some magical birth powder over that village that night.

"I can't take it anymore, get it out of me!"

She screamed this over and over again, begging for a C-section, hitting herself and pulling her sister by the hair. The epidural she had been given wasn't really affecting her and she was somewhere between hysteria and despair after an hour with full dilation and no progress.

And us? We encouraged and comforted her, and told her that she actually can take it, and that if she would only push this would all end. But she did not want to push, only to shout that she couldn't take it anymore. In the end she had a C-section, after three and a half hours of full dilation.

In the end, it turned out that she was right and we were just thick. She really couldn't do it – the baby had entered the pelvis in a crooked way and in the occipital posterior position. When he was born, his head looked like the head of King Tut - a bit elongated and tilted to the side, a sign of the last few hours, during which the head had been pressed through the birth canal.

It made me think about this whole business of "yes you can" that we use so much. I was reminded of my own birth, during which I had pushed for three and a half hours, and because of the baby's position, I too was unable to give birth. When they told me, "Yes you can," I knew that I just couldn't and it frustrated me, terribly.

But how do you know which woman is just saying that she can't and which really can't? Sometimes there are doctors or midwives who give a woman a long lecture about how she can make it, and how she will never become a mother if she can't pull herself together and push. They talk about positive thinking, and feed her all kinds of admonitions and exhortations. I too sometimes sin by having these kinds of thoughts about the women here.

I had a woman in labor that simply didn't want to push, but also didn't want a vacuum or to undergo surgery. She only wanted her mother to take her home and for the birth to be over. She kept begging, "Oh mother! Enough already, enough already!" And to the doctor she screamed, "Do something! I don't want to give birth, it hurts! It hurts me so! Stop it!" The doctor kindly told her that he was sorry but it really was not up to him, it was not he who invented the way in which women give birth, and this was how it has been going on for millions of years.

It's true that women have been giving birth this way for millions of years and before that there were zebras and giraffes who delivered their young without any problems, but in the last few centuries we have lost it a little; we've lost the ability to give birth alone, to trust our bodies to know how to breathe, how to move, how to push. We have grown too accustomed to doctors and midwives checking on us to know if we have even started labor; to help us when we are in pain; to cut our perineum so the baby will come out; to give us permission to hold our baby or feed him; to allow us to get out of bed and go home. We forgot that our body is smarter, that our programming is divine, and that the responsibility for our bodies and our children is solely ours. By the way, in the end that woman was convinced that there was no other way, gave one long push, and the baby was out.

Another woman suddenly started screaming that she knows, deep down inside, that something is going to go seriously wrong and begged for a C-section, and said that she knew herself and her body and that please, please, please, we must believe her. In our ward, we do not have C-sections without a medical reason, and in this case there really was no reason. But the woman was so mesmerizing in her deep inner conviction, it caused even her physician,

Dr. Sophie, who is usually the most logical person imaginable, to begin having doubts.

Fortunately, while Dr. Sophie contemplated the matter and consulted with the head physician, the woman had already delivered vaginally a nice healthy baby.

I thought a lot about what happened in that birth. How do you know what to do, and what would have happened if something had gone wrong; and what would have happened, on the other hand, if she had undergone a C-section and something had gone wrong with the operation? How can you know? How can you really know?

I still walk around with a smile on my inner face

Sunday morning is usually a day of inductions, elective C-sections and a lot of women that come to our reception desk after having rested at home during the Sabbath. But yesterday it was raining and the beginning of the shift was quiet.

When I arrived to my shift there was only one woman in the ward, having her tenth birth. She was there the whole night and her birth was progressing slowly, just like first-time mothers - the womb was a little tired, what can you do? She had painful contractions but she didn't suffer from it. It turns out that pain does not have to be automatically translated into suffering.

The mother, an Ultra-Orthodox Jewish woman, constantly thanked everyone or prayed really hard. Her husband, who was long-bearded and bright-eyed, prayed in the corner, hardly speaking a word, but giving out a little smile. When I met her, she had been with a 9 centimeter dilation for the last two hours. Her waters had not broken yet, but the head was very high in the cervix, so they did not try to break them for fear of complications with the umbilical cord.[45] So we waited. During rounds, the doctor examined

---

45 A few words about umbilical cord prolapse - in most births, the first part of the baby to be born into this world is the head, followed by the body and the umbilical cord. Sometimes there is a situation in which the umbilical cord precedes the head and drops through the vagina. The risk factors for umbilical cord prolapse are: Polyhydramnios, spontaneous breaking of waters, or breech presentation. If the prolapse occurs it may endanger the life of the baby, because the pressure generated on the umbilical cord compromises its blood supply. When identifying an umbilical cord prolapse, the person

her and said that now the head had descended enough to break the waters. She said, "They always break my waters," so he broke her waters and continued his round. Meanwhile, I just wore gloves and waited. It was clear that she would give birth really soon.

"Do you feel any pressure?" I asked.

"Not yet."

Another minute passed. "Is there any pressure?"

"No...Actually, yes!!!"

And in a flash the head was out and was followed by the body. Wow, that was fast. After so many births that progressed at a slow pace and women with epidurals who pushed and pushed without anything getting pushed out; after all that, bang, the baby was out. It was so beautiful.

But the most beautiful thing about this birth happened after that. The woman and the man were so happy. She called out, "A miracle! It's a miracle! God made a miracle!" Despite having given birth nine times already, she didn't take anything for granted and saw this new birth as a miraculous event. It was so inspiring to see the excitement and love this little girl met as she entered this world.

After this birth, the rain stopped and the reception desk began to fill up with people. At one point I was called to the delivery room to monitor a woman who had been admitted and, due to lack of space in reception, had gone straight to the delivery room. The moment I walked in, I immediately recognized her - I had delivered her when I was still an intern in my midwifery course. She also

---

who examined the woman must keep his or her fingers in the vagina and try to push the baby's head so as not to press on the cord, while preparing the woman for an emergency C-section. The fear of umbilical cord prolapse is one of the reasons why it is recommended for women whose waters have broken to go immediately to a hospital, even if contractions haven't started yet.

remembered me and we were both very happy. She told me that her waters had broken during the night and that she was in labor now. Of course she refused a vaginal examination or ultrasound. After all, she hadn't undergone any tests during her whole pregnancy, so why spoil it by starting now?

You have to understand, a woman who comes to give birth must show proof that she has started her labor or that her waters have broken, but I knew her and I knew that she knows her body well and that she knows when it was in labor and when it was just sending a false alarm. So I immediately got her admitted and when I called the doctor, who in this case was the head of the delivery room, to complete her medical admission, he was a bit mad at me:

"What is her PV?" he barked. Translation: "What are the findings of her vaginal examination?"

"I don't know," I replied.

"How do we know her waters broke?"

"Because she said so," I replied.

"And how do we know she is really in labor?" He pressed.

"Because she says so and I believe her."

"How do we know the baby is not in breech position?"

"Ahhhhh..." I hesitated, "Maybe we can palpate the belly and find out this way?"

"Well, I agree. I have no problem with that. What about the baby's weight?"

At this point the woman intervened in the conversation and said she thought the baby weighs seven and a half pounds, according to her experience from previous pregnancies. Her estimation was accepted. The whole weight estimation by ultrasound is quite dubious anyway. A study in which three fetal weight assessment methods were compared - ultrasound, weight assessment by feeling the woman's abdomen and the woman's assessment, provided that it was not her first pregnancy - showed that in terms of accuracy the most reliable is the woman's own assessment; after that, feeling the abdomen, and ultrasound last of all. It happens to us a lot that we make decisions based on weight estimations that were made by ultrasound, and after the delivery it turns out we were not even close.

Two weeks ago, for example, we received a delivery that was induced due to suspicion of intrauterine growth retardation. The estimated fetal weight was about 5 lb, 8 oz. In the end, a cute little teddy bear, weighing 8 lb, 6 oz was born. At the end of the delivery the doctor said, "We have to stop relying so much on that ultrasound!" And to that I add: "Amen!" Nowadays, when you ask this doctor about weight estimations he says with a smile, "Six and a half, give or take a couple of pounds. I'm 99% sure..." It teaches us that doctors are also aware of the limitations of ultrasound scans. By the way, the further the weight is from the average fetal weight in either direction, so too the margin of error increases. So, weight estimation is just as the name suggests; only an estimation.

Anyway, let's get back to our story. We were left alone and as I knew her from her previous birth, I didn't try to offer her anything she did not want. She was wearing the same plaid dress from last time, with the same socks and shoes - this is probably her regular delivery outfit - and just stood quietly by the bed. I remembered that she had been that composed even at the height of her labor, so I asked her to just tell me when she is about to deliver.

After a few minutes she said, "It's coming," and then climbed onto the bed, as she didn't want to use the delivery chair this time. I connected the monitor, and then she announced solemnly, "Here it comes."

I wore gloves and watched calmly as her baby girl was born. Afterwards, I put her on her mother's tummy and, as with her sibling in the previous birth, she immediately began to nurse. It all happened so quietly. Fifteen minutes later, I went out to consult with another midwife regarding the integrity of the placenta and everyone was amazed: "What? She gave birth already? We didn't hear anything." The weight, by the way, was off by only three ounces from the woman's assessment. Do I need to add more?

Now, my inner smile and I are going to sleep.

Out of sight, out of mind

Yesterday I was asked to help for a few hours in the nursery. I went with a heavy heart, and sure enough, there I found crying, screaming, yelling babies whose mothers were in some other place; the veteran nurses no longer heard their crying. To them, a crying baby is a healthy and alert baby, and that's enough. "I'm much more concerned about those who do not cry," admitted one of the older nurses. "I at least know that those who cry are breathing."

Unlike them, this crying really gets to me, touching some exposed nerve endings. It holds me there, cuts me and tears me from the inside. It was always that way, but now that I was a mother, it had become even worse. I tried to rock the cradles, to talk and sing; at one point I had enough time to pick up a baby and act as a substitute mother for him, even if just for ten minutes, until he fell asleep. And while I was talking to him and stroking him, another baby started crying, and I tried to convey to her in telepathy, since we are not permitted to walk around with a baby in our hands, that I would soon be with her. Then we received a new baby from the delivery room, who just lay alone in his plastic box, his hand holding onto a tube that was hanging there next to him.

At five in the afternoon, the babies who are not rooming in, which is the vast majority of them, go out to visit their mothers. They can stay with their mothers until eight at night, but at six, some of the mothers are already returning their newborns to the nursery.

I really don't understand those mothers who do not ask themselves what happens when their baby stays without them in the nursery; or their families, who sell them this nonsense that they should rest after birth and that they can relax without the baby; or the system that makes it all possible, and even encourages it, rather than taking a stand and saying that really only sick infants should be in the nursery, and all the rest should be with their mothers. They could even back up this option, for example, by having an assistant to help mothers take care of their babies when they are alone and tired. Being alone with a baby after birth is really difficult, if not impossible, especially if you have had a long and difficult labor or a C-section.

Then I went to visit the NICU. Most premature babies there were really tiny – from twenty to thirty ounces, and one can hardly see them among all the surrounding tubes and paraphernalia. Some were sleeping, perhaps dreaming that they were still in the womb, growing slowly; and some were dying, with varying degrees of brain damage. One baby, the last survivor of triplets who were born in their twenty-fourth week, was in a bad and unstable state. In the background, there was no sound other than the bleeping noises of the monitors, occasionally interrupted by the pumping sound of the respirator. Worst of all was the absence of parents. Out of all seven preemies in care, only one mother came during my shift to pump some breast milk for her baby.

It is hard to know why this is so. Luckily, I haven't delivered prematurely and never personally experienced the ordeal of a baby's prolonged hospitalization in intensive care, sometimes with other children still waiting at home. In my estimation, much of the problem lies with a system that doesn't really encourage parents to be with their children. How lovely it would be if there was a bed for the parent next to each baby, or at least an easy chair, where one could stay comfortably for hours, and with screens between the beds, to enable breastfeeding in privacy.

In our NICU, there is one room that has sofas and armchairs and coffee and TV, and one can stay there alone, or with one's premature baby, if he does not need to be connected to oxygen or any medical devices. And still, I see that we could encourage even more parental contact, and resist ejecting parents from the room so often. By the way, I think this is a general problem with hospitalization in intensive care, and these same issues bothered me when I was in nursing school, in adult intensive care.

Throughout my shift, I wanted to escape from the nursery. I wanted to cry, and to run to the maternity ward and call out to all the mothers, "Your babies are crying and screaming in the nursery! Quick, go take them now!". I wanted to take the babies home with me; I wanted to breastfeed the ones who were crying; I wanted to return home to my daughter and kiss her a million times and hold her tightly and never leave her.

But instead, I stayed. I did not scream and I did not cry. I comforted the babies as best I could, stroking them and explaining to them what was happening, because I believe they understand everything at this age - if not the words, than at least the intent. In truth, this is not just a sentimental belief of a breastfeeding mother with milk dripping from her ears. More and more studies in this area show that babies do understand, do remember, do experience these times in the nursery as hard times. These first hours are a critical period in our lives, a period of imprinting; and all of these early experiences to a large extent form the way we view the world. It's a bit like ducklings, who think that the first creature they set eyes on after hatching from the egg, is their mother; and so if they happen to see a person instead, then they will follow that person instead. To think that a baby does not experience fear or pain, that he does not feel lonely or miss his mother, is just not true.

At the end of the shift, I walked with heavy steps back home. At night, while I was kissing Ya'ara a million times, holding her tightly and nursing her, I dreamed I was back in this sad place. The next morning I awoke, still full of pain from the dream and, with no outlet for it, finding it hard to contain it all.

Why not start earlier?

A midwife friend told me once that she had given a lecture about birth to children in fourth and fifth grades, and asked them to draw a picture of a woman in childbirth. They all drew a woman lying in a hospital bed. That means that even at this young age, the idea is already rooted in their minds, probably because of what they see on TV and read in books.

Many times, I think that during childbirth, it's too late; too late to explain, too late to tutor. How do you explain something to a woman who is discovering that her concept of "the most painful thing I've ever experienced" is changing every few minutes? When we get women to consent to an epidural, they laugh and say they are ready to sign a mortgage if that what it takes; they do not care for explanations right now, they just want the pain to go away.

After each birth, I ask the woman if she wants rooming in. Some ask me for my opinion and then say they want rooming in, but in practice, I see that most end up giving up on that idea, probably after their mothers advise them to rest a bit because, "If you do not rest now, when will you?"

I have a dream of giving one of those birth preparation courses to twelve-year-olds. Well, not a "real" birth preparation course but something that would open the door to an otherwise unfamiliar world and provide an alternative to everything they see in the movies. I tested this idea today on about eleven girls who go to school in my community. They are now having two weeks of separate classes for boys and girls, in which they discuss subjects such as adolescence, sexuality, relationships between boys and girls and so on. I was asked to teach a class and of course I chose a subject that is close to my heart: Birth.

I started with the exercise that my friend had given me, and asked each one to draw a woman giving birth. This led to a wave of protests, "But what should I draw exactly?" or, "How should I know what it looks like?" and so on. But after two minutes, all the girls were busy drawing, and after fifteen minutes it was hard to stop them.

We sat in a circle on the carpet and I asked them what birth actually is. I asked them to explain it through their drawings. I was fascinated to see what they produced, and discovered that indeed, by seventh grade, it is already too late. All of their pictures depicted women in the hospital, all lying on a bed. One drawing showed the lithotomy position (feet raised apart); another showed the husband waiting outside. Someone drew only the mother's face, which was completely terrified, and another drew a cartoon, with the mother shouting, "*Aahahhahahahah.*" The woman was holding her husband's hand and a thought bubble showed him thinking, "Why do I deserve this?" And by the way, that girl is the daughter of a midwife...

I tried to ask each girl who presented a picture to explain the meaning behind it, and to share what else she knows about birth. For example, I asked the girl who painted the woman in the lithotomy position how long, in her opinion, the woman had been lying like that; and I asked the girl who painted the husband outside the room why was he out there and whether he was allowed to enter.

The girls were excited, open, and highly enthusiastic. This age is so confusing; one can actually see on their faces the emotions, thoughts and hormones that are storming within. How hard it must be - I wouldn't go back to this age for all the fortune in the world.

Next I asked them what, in their opinion, a woman in childbirth does, and that developed into interesting discussion. I had more questions, but I wasn't able to ask them, because they bombarded me with questions of their own: what are these waters that break, what is the placenta attached to, why do some women have a C-section, and a hundred others. They also wanted to tell about the births of their siblings, about how they themselves came into the world, or about shows they had seen on television...

Finally, we watched a film about a natural birth that takes place in the home of Naoli, a very special woman from Mexico, who is a midwife herself. I felt that it planted some very good seeds in them about the idea of a natural birth at home, in water, in the presence of the husband and family. It's not that I think that this is the only way to give birth, and certainly it is not right for every woman, but at least I tried to balance the image created by all those stupid films and TV shows. In the movies, the woman is always sitting relaxed in a restaurant or on a plane, holding her belly, when suddenly she starts screaming in a terrified voice, "Help, the baby is coming!" And then, within two minutes, she starts to push and give birth, on the restaurant table, of course, with the waitress acting as her midwife.

It's hard to believe how much trouble these Hollywood films cause. Many women call for an ambulance upon feeling the first contraction, and a lot of couples who are filled with anticipation for the birth to take place, do not understand why it ends up taking so long when for Claire, the blonde girl from the "Lost" series, it took only ten minutes. They are sure that something is terribly wrong with their birth and no explanation I give them eases their minds.

I began to envision giving such a course to kindergarten children, but my neighbor, who is a kindergarten teacher, burst my bubble, telling me that the Ministry of Education in Israel does not allow anything to do with sex, death or God to be taught in kindergarten.

"Whaaaat?" I cried, when I heard that. What was left to talk about then?

Stretching the limits of what's possible

I'll begin by informing you that the mother and baby are safe and well. Now, that being said, something happened yesterday that happens once in a thousand C-sections or so; that is, every two and a half to three years in our delivery room. And yet, when it happens, it rattles everyone completely.

So here it goes. She was a woman giving birth for the third time. She insisted on having an epidural when she was dilated only two and a half centimeters, and after the epidural, she felt good, the birth progressed smoothly and everyone was happy. That is, until she reached 6 centimeters dilation and all progress stopped. From then on, things started to go wrong. In addition to the lack of progress, FHR decelerations began to appear; nothing serious, but a situation that requires some attention.

It was something of a Catch 22: On the one hand, we wanted to strengthen her contractions with Pitocin, but because of the FHR decelerations with each contraction, we couldn't. On the other hand, the delivery was not progressing and we couldn't drag things on forever, in part because there were FHR decelerations. After some time passed, in which the decelerations continued and the birth did not progress, we suggested to the woman that we end her delivery by C-section, but she refused. Then the heart rate decelerations intensified and were considered so severe as to be a very good reason to perform a C-section if birth did not occur in an hour; nevertheless she did not want to go to surgery under any circumstances.

It went on like this for six hours - six hours with a dilation of 6 centimeters and with no progress. While it is true that childbirth is not an exact science and every woman is different, six hours with no progress at this stage is a very abnormal situation.

We tried to do everything to progress the delivery: change positions, press certain pressure points, let her move around and whatnot, but her dilation stayed the same. It later turned out that the baby had entered the birth canal completely lopsided and, even though he was really tiny, could not go through. This is very typical for births in which the woman received an epidural relatively early.

So, after two hours with no progress, we suggested to her, according to the procedure, that she have a C-section…but she refused.

After three hours with no progress, we were really pressing for surgery…but she refused.

After four hours, we pleaded and explained the risk of a prolonged labor that did not progress…but she refused.

After five hours, we recruited more and more doctors and everyone in turn tried to speak to her heart…but she refused.

After six hours (and let me remind you – there had been serious and frightening decelerations in pulse for six hours now and there was no progress in the labor) the hospital director came and had a heart-to-heart with her and… she finally agreed to surgery.

We ran into the operating theater, where a tiny baby was born looking not that good at first -- pale and panting -- but after a few minutes, it seemed that he was recovering well. An hour after the surgery, the woman began to bleed, drastically, and the bleeding did not stop.

It went on, and on and on. She received blood transfusions and plasma equal to the volume of her blood, twice. She was admitted to intensive care and underwent more surgery in an attempt to stop the bleeding. Her uterus simply did not contract after surgery and the massive bleeding did not stop. That's what happens sometimes after a very long birth with no progress. The uterus gets tired, losing its ability to contract properly, and when it does not contract, the blood vessels that were attached to the placenta simply continue to bleed. In the third and final surgery, they removed her uterus; there was no other choice.

There is something in the perception of a hysterectomy for a woman still in her prime that is so... I don't even know how to define it. When I heard it, I couldn't believe it, and neither could anyone else. And yes, it happens sometimes, it even happened to one of our midwives, but when you confront it yourself in real life, it's totally different.

I don't have any incredible insights about this, but I just want to talk about it, because I think part of me still can't digest it.

And the woman shouts: "Joseph! What have you done to me?"

Basically, this is just a myth. At least I have never heard a woman screaming at her husband, "What have you done to me!" during birth. They scream a lot of other things; they beg for the labor to be over, for the pain to go away; they call for their mothers; they cry for their dads; they ask God to do something; and they ask the baby to get out already. Sometimes it's funny, sometimes it's scary, and sometimes your heart just breaks.

One woman, for example, repeatedly screamed, "Dana! Do something! Why don't you help me?" She shouted this in a very loud voice, so that everyone on our floor heard her (I don't know about the other floors, but I have my suspicions). And I actually did help her; it was just that her baby was about to come out, and the epidural was not having much effect at this point. I'm afraid that all of the people who heard her thought, why the hell doesn't Dana help that poor woman begging for assistance? What kind of a midwife is she anyway?

Another woman screamed just as loudly, "My twat's on fire! My twat's on fire!" and all the other people in the delivery room were happy when she finally gave birth and ended their embarrassment.

On the other hand, there are women who tell great jokes during labor. It is not clear how, but in between contractions they have such great quips that afterwards I'm sorry I didn't write them down. There are other women who ask the same questions over and over, again and again. I explain at length, making sure they understand, and five minutes later they ask the same question again. I fight the urge to get angry and remind myself that it's usually a sign of anxiety. Instead, I try to focus on caressing and smiling and, surprisingly, their questions gradually cease.

Some women are just quiet and do not say anything. When asked how they are doing, they do not respond; when they are in pain they do not cry, but rather close up even more, terrifyingly reserved. Those women scare me a little, because I sometimes wonder what's going on in there - pleasant and peaceful composure or a dance of fears and inner demons.

There are women who bless everything. In Judaism it is believed that at birth, a mother's prayers are always answered, so many religious women at birth pray for other women who have never given birth and who long for a child. It is quite moving to see a woman who, throughout her contractions, is simultaneously praying and begging for the health and happiness of other women. And I'm there, next to them, and they almost always bless me in the same breath with their fellow friends and family members. They ask the name of my mother and pray for me to have sons, although I actually would not mind having a few more daughters, and they pray for my health, longevity and happiness; and I think to myself that after being blessed with all this wealth and health, my prayer can only be one of thanks.

More about judgment

As I wrote earlier, one of the hardest things for me as a midwife, not to mention as a person, is to refrain from judgment; to completely accept another person without trying to change her or thinking that I know what's best for her. Despite my difficulty with this, I do believe I'm making progress.

Here is a story for illustration:

A few days ago, a woman came in with a stillborn baby, a very, very sad situation. It was the first boy after five girls, and they had all been waiting for him. Of course, it would have been just as sad if it had been a girl. The condition had been initially diagnosed in her HMO clinic and received further confirmation in the hospital. The woman now had to begin the long and tedious process of labor induction, knowing that there would be no living infant at the end. Two days after her arrival, the husband spoke with their rabbi, who told him it was not true that the baby had died and that we should connect a monitor and see that he is actually alive. The husband and wife were filled with hope, which unfortunately was proven wrong. The baby really was dead.

When I heard that, I almost screamed in anger. What a stupid and arrogant rabbi. Was it not hard enough to undergo this ordeal; did he really need to add to their misery a strong dosage of shattered hopes and dreams? Why did this woman deserve to undergo another painful emotional upheaval? And then I thought, *Oh, those fools, why did they even ask the advice of such a Rabbi! Can't they decide anything on their own, can't they think for themselves?*

Then, remembering my decision to avoid judging others, I said to myself, *If I think that it is best for them to think just like me, than basically I'm trying to deny them the right to think for themselves.* Perhaps what's best is for everyone to take responsibility for themselves, and if they feel the need, for example, to ask the advice of a rabbi (even one who is an idiot), then it's their right. About the rabbi, well, I still have not found a way not to judge him. Maybe next year I will succeed in becoming even more understanding. I definitely see it as something to strive for. In the delivery room, I encounter the results of many consultations with rabbis and often I feel like pulling out some hair - my own and the rabbi's. I once saw twins die because of a rabbi's bad advice, and I've witnessed the death of a few infants, following the advice of non-Jewish religious leaders of all kinds; it drives me crazy.

By the way, even though it drives me crazy, I try to go with the flow. Once I even contributed some of my milk to a woman whose rabbi told her to drink mother's milk as a sort of talisman for a successful birth. It did not work. In the end, she gave birth by C-section.

Falling in love with first births

Many midwives prefer to attend repeated births, because in most cases they are much easier than first-time births. It is usually less painful for the woman, the delivery progresses faster, they push once or twice and it's done, the woman breastfeeds easily and everything just flows. First-time births, on the other hand, can sometimes seem to go on forever.

After attending a series of first births, however, I suddenly fell in love. I fell in love with the wonders of a perineum that gets dilated for the first time. It happens so slowly, but it's such a wonder - one of the Seven Wonders of the World, in my opinion. Bit by bit, millimeter by millimeter, and suddenly the baby's head is crowning. And though it seemed like it would never happen, never, at some point, it does. The head comes out and the body follows. The woman becomes a mother for the first time and it's so beautiful. I fell in love with the entire experience.

One of those first births this week was just terrible. Actually, it was not the birth itself that was terrible, but that one of the new mother's family members, probably her sister-in-law, just didn't want me there. She thought I was some unprofessional midwife, because I wouldn't yell at the woman to push when she was 5 centimeters dilated. Of course you're not supposed to push before you reach full dilation of 10 centimeters... She wanted me to massage the perineum right from the beginning of labor, even before there was any dilation, something that would do no good, but would have caused a terrible edema. She wanted me to lift the woman's legs up like they did thirty years ago, although it's very uncomfortable. She was unsatisfied because I didn't yell at the woman, "Push! Push!"

really loudly and because I didn't want to check her progress every fifteen minutes or so; in short, because of the terrible midwife that I am.

At some point, she said something about how her relative needed more professional help than what I was providing. Ugh! I wanted to throw my gloves in her face and leave. But I didn't, and instead I struggled to smile despite the humiliation, so that I could stay with the woman. But one of the most important – and most difficult - things for a midwife to know, in my opinion, is when to do nothing. And here I was being challenged by a woman who didn't understand, and simply could not accept, that sometimes the best course of action is to take no action.

The next day made up for it. Despite the fact that when I got there, the woman's mother had a sour face and was already threatening to go to another hospital, and the woman giving birth seemed cranky and angry herself, I swore that last evening's incident would not repeat itself. I gave the mother and her daughter a nice pep talk. I told them about first births, that it's natural for it to take some time and that it actually allows the body to ready itself at its own pace, without pressure. I told them how important it is to try and stay cheerful during labor and not to think that if you feel pain it's a sign that something terrible has happened. On the contrary, it is a sign that something good has happened and that the delivery has progressed. I talked about how pain doesn't necessarily mean suffering, and that it actually only hurts during the contractions and that in between you can rest and gather your strength. As I spoke, I saw the expression of the woman softening and then her whole body relaxed. Her mother began to nod as well; reluctant nods initially, but later, ones full of energy and delight.

So we became an inseparable team for the rest of the birth, which was very challenging. It was a first birth with a long and painful latent phase, a husband on his way from Jerusalem getting live updates from the delivery room and an epidural shot that didn't arrive due to a shortage of anesthesiologists... nevertheless, from the mother's initial scowls and the suffering face of the woman giving birth, we reached a state of relaxed sleep in between contractions, smiles of joy and the amazing ability to cope during the labor itself.

Over the next hour, she progressed from 5 to 10 centimeters dilation and did just great. Even her mother gave her amazing support, the likes of which I haven't seen in a long while. We had such fun together and it was such a 180 degree turnaround from the day before, that even my ego managed to fully recover – especially after the fiftieth time that they said I was *an angel/ Just great, the best!* and so on.

I was glad that she ended up having a good experience, despite the not-so-promising start, and I was glad that I had chosen to make an effort, rather than just retreating into my shell and complaining about all the unkind people in my care. This is how it goes in a delivery room; you can experience a journey of personal development *and* be fully present during births. What fun it is!

They could make a movie about this

It was 5 AM when the woman arrived to give birth at our hospital. She was a refugee from Sudan, with coal black skin and partially bleached braids, and very beautiful. She did not understand a word of Hebrew, or English for that matter, and she was very scared and very much opposed to anyone touching her. This was her fourth birth, but it seemed that her previous births had not taken place in a hospital, and so she had many scars that hadn't healed properly. Her entrance was turbulent and wild, and so we skipped the reception desk and went straight into the delivery room. She was almost at the end of her labor.

I was taking care of another woman, or rather four other women, so the other midwife on duty, who was also looking after several women, took her under her care. The midwife was Olivia, an African-born Nigerian woman; beautiful with chocolate milk skin and bleached purple braids.

I thought to myself, *how did two women from Africa, who traveled so far from home, happen to meet in a remote Israeli hospital delivery room?* The world acts in mysterious ways. Just the word "Africa" touches something deep in my soul. Africa. Africa. Africa. I immediately get a vision of a Savannah, dusty acacia trees, a leopard stretching and yawning on a branch, and beautiful women wearing colorful decorative beads, walking with their heads high. Africa.

Two African women meet in an Israeli delivery room. They do not find any common language, despite the fact that Olivia knows five African languages; apparently these are not the right five. The levels of anxiety rise, both for the woman and the midwife, who detects signs of HELLP syndrome, which is somewhat similar to preeclampsia but far more dangerous. Olivia tries to explain to the mother the need for all kinds of tests. In the room, there's a lot of fear, shouting, crying and confusion; and above all, the frustration that comes when you can't communicate at all.

In the end, after she had finished giving birth, someone realized that the woman also spoke Arabic, so guess whom they called to translate? That's right, me.

Once in a lifetime

Every birth is different; a unique event like nothing that has been before and nothing that will ever happen in the future, and with each birth you can learn something new - about yourself, about other people or even about other midwives... if only you let yourself learn.

Yesterday, I took care of a woman giving birth for the third time, who wanted a natural birth, the same as her previous ones. After a short monitor check-up at reception, she went into the bathroom and was there for an hour or more. At this point we met. I introduced myself and asked her to enter the room, so we could listen to the fetal heartbeat over the monitor.

She was a beautiful woman with long red hair, who felt comfortable with nudity and she preferred to stay naked for the entire birth - just my kind of woman. After listening to the fetus's heartbeat over the monitor for a few minutes, she decided to relax a bit in a chair; just a regular hospital chair with a backrest and arms. Perhaps an armchair is a more accurate name.

During contractions, she would lean forward, and her husband and I would massage her back; in between contractions, she would sit back and rest. At some point, I went to eat, telling her first that if she felt any pressure, she should call me. Upon finishing my sandwich, I suddenly saw the green light that says *nurse required* flashing next to their room. I rushed into the room and the woman said she felt really intense pressure.

I asked her where she wanted to give birth and she said that she didn't really know, but since she was sitting comfortably in a chair, it seemed silly to move her to the bed. I arranged a comfortable birth station for us -- a small mattress in front, a dry cloth in hand and a pad to absorb liquids -- and we waited. During her next contraction, her waters broke in a huge gush. Luckily they were clean, because they soaked me from head to toe. Then she said that she felt the pressure decreasing. I explained to her that this was natural and that her uterus was just preparing for a big, strong contraction. I have noticed that after a big break between contractions, during the second stage of birth, there is usually a strong and effective contraction. And sure enough, during the next contraction she felt intense pressure again. She moved to the edge of the chair and slowly the head came out, and after it the body, and all I had to do was grab the baby and lift it up to her.

Immediately after the baby was born, the mother leaned back in the chair. I was finally convinced that this armchair was absolutely ideal for birth; much more comfortable than our official birthing chair. Everything was so lovely, quiet, dark and cozy. And she was so pretty, oh so pretty!

Then we had the placenta to attend to. In her two previous births the mother had experienced problems with placentas that did not separate, or did not separate entirely. This time, the same thing happened. Even though the placenta did separate naturally, a part remained inside the uterus and we had to go into the operation room to remove it manually. But because of the great harmony and peace that filled the delivery room, everything went quietly and smoothly, without any stress and without unnecessary excitement. Perhaps it was also like that because the same thing had happened to her before. Either way, part of her was expecting it to happen and so she prepared herself for it. At the end of this process, she returned to nurse her baby as if they had never parted. It felt complete and undisturbed.

I spoke to her after the birth and she said she had felt very good during the delivery - that she felt she could do whatever she wanted and had not been limited by anything. Funny, but I felt that way, too. Often the barriers are in our minds; the fear of delivering in a strange position that I have no experience with, or fear of doing something I'm not used to. This time I did not feel these inhibitions and felt as if it had loosened up a few other things within me. The experience created openness and flexibility for other births in the future.

After this birth, a song was born from within me:

She dances her birth dance
With great big eyes and a great big body
With great power within
With great power within

She dances her life dance
And the song of the child that has yet to see the light
Plays within

She dances her birth dance
In circles
Spinning
Giving herself

She dances her birth dance
With no crowd, no choreographer
With only God
Watching and listening

"Hello, I'm here to give birth, I think"

This is a quite common opening phrase heard at our reception desk, and the women who say it usually look just like the one in front of me: freshly showered, their wet hair meticulously brushed, with a bit of makeup and jewelry on and looking very relaxed. In fact, the woman doesn't really look like she is about to give birth, she looks like she is about to go out to a café or the cinema.

When I ask her husband to go down and sign her in with the admissions office, he replies in a tense and nervous voice, "But I don't want to miss the birth!"

"Don't worry," I say to calm him down. "I think there is plenty of time, and it only takes five minutes to go down to the office."

"But she's in real pain. At home she had contractions every five minutes!" he presses on and a bit of hysteria sneaks into his voice.

The woman joins in and says, "It's true! Here, right now, for example, I'm having a very painful contraction. See?"

I look at her during her contraction. She is calm and smiling, her body is relaxed, she doesn't move an inch or breathe heavily, and during her contraction she continues to tell me how long she's been having these contractions and how much they hurt. I'm not terribly impressed with how painful her contractions are, and the husband notices and tells me, "Don't look at her that way, she is very strong. She can suffer terrible pain and it won't show at all."

And the woman agrees, "I really have a very high pain threshold!"

"Okay," I concede, even though in my heart I'm still not terribly impressed. I check the woman and discover, to her complete astonishment, that she has no dilation, no shortening of the cervix, no nothing.

"But she's been having really painful contractions for the last half an hour..." the husband tries to convince me for the last time.

This is the so-called latent phase[46] - the beginning of birth or maybe just false contractions. In most cases, midwives can estimate a woman's dilation quite well by looking at her face, her demeanor during the contraction, the way she walks, the sounds she makes, and in particular, how she acts when she is having a contraction. Is she talkative and extroverted (latent phase) or does she look like someone closed-up in her own private world, not really *with us* so to speak (active labor)? It's not really an exact science, of course, but many times it's pretty accurate.

Later, another woman comes in. It is her first pregnancy and she is here for a routine visit at week forty. I examine her. "So unnecessary," Dana the midwife mutters to herself, "it's clear that she is not in labor. Who needs those vaginal exams anyway?" And then, to my astonishment, I find that she is 8 centimeters dilated! I remind myself that there are those rare and lucky women who don't feel any pain during childbirth...

This, for me, is a lesson in humility.

---

46 A few words about the stages of birth: Birth is divided into three stages and the first stage of labor is divided into two phases. The latent phase of birth may take anywhere from several hours to several days and is characterized by short, irregular and not very painful contractions, at least in most cases. The latent phase leads to a dilation of three to four centimeters. The active phase usually lasts several hours; dilation progresses faster - an average of one to one and a half centimeters of dilation an hour – and includes long, painful contractions in constant intervals. Towards the end of the active phase, progress is usually quite rapid and turbulent, and this phase is called the transition phase. The active phase ends with full dilation. The second stage begins with full dilation and ends with the baby's delivery. This is a stage of strong contractions, where the woman begins to feel the need to push out the baby. Sometimes there is a full dilation but the baby is still relatively high up the canal and the woman does not feel any need to push. In this case, she should wait until she feels pressure. The third stage of labor begins after the delivery, ends with the birth of the placenta, and usually takes several minutes.

If at first you don't succeed

I want to write about a very moving birth I attended. This woman is also a friend of mine; not a very close friend, but still dear to my heart. We used to work together in the Pediatrics Department and when she arrived two years ago, to give birth for the first time, I just so happened to be there. That birth began with an induction, due to the baby's weight being estimated as very high. The induction led to an early epidural, which probably led to the baby's occipital posterior presentation, and finally, after three or four hours at 9 centimeters dilation, the doctors decided to perform a C-section. The baby was indeed quite big – nine and a half pounds, if I remember correctly.

And now, she was about to give birth for the second time. Since there had been several complications in surgery during her first birth and some problems afterwards with breastfeeding, she very much wanted to have a natural birth. I had bumped into her at work a few days earlier, and she had shared with me her hopes for a natural birth, but I thought she probably didn't want me there after the whole ordeal with her previous birth. But, when I arrived on this morning to the delivery room, she was there, all cheerful and happy to see me, saying, "How great, I was hoping you'd be here!"

Her waters had broken at home and yet she had experienced almost no contractions. Weight estimation predicted that the baby would be between eight and a half and nine pounds. At our hospital, we recommend a repeat C-section in such a case, but the doctor was honest and told her that there had been a new directive from the Ministry of Health, recommending a repeat C-section only when the baby is over nine pounds, fifteen ounces. He tried to estimate her chance of giving birth vaginally with some birth calculator website on the Internet that incorporates all kind of variables and gives the chance of success. Her score was 46% for a successful vaginal birth -- depressing! Her spirit was crushed and she seriously considered having surgery. I explained to her that this website does not include the really important variables, such as her motivation or the support of the people around her and so on, and we agreed that surgery is always an option we can fall back on.

The most important thing to do was to avoid an early epidural, which was probably what had arrested her previous birth. I also encouraged her by saying that her belly looked smaller compared to her previous birth. Soon she began to have contractions, and after about an hour of showers and massages, she said that was it, she couldn't take it anymore and she wanted an epidural. She started to say all kinds of things, like how weak she was and why was her pain threshold so low and how she should really be stronger.

I want to say something about this. So many women beat themselves up for having a low pain threshold. Even if we disregard for a minute the conditions that make it hard to cope with contractions, such as the continuous monitoring that limits movement, being outside of one's natural environment and so on, there are still women that just have a lower pain threshold. And I say, so what? So you have low endurance. Does it make you a bad mother? Does it mean you are a bad person? Out of all the important attributes a person could have, I can think of a hundred qualities far more important than being able to endure pain, such as being generous, caring, patient, loving, funny, sensitive, peaceful and much more. So you don't have a high pain threshold, so what?

Unfortunately I get to see quite a few women who make it their mission to have a *natural birth* and in the end they ask us to take the baby to the nursery right afterwards, because they have no energy left to be with her after a long and painful labor; but hey, who cares - at least they showed endurance. As you know, I'm obviously not against natural childbirth, quite the opposite, but why should a woman torture and torment herself and feel that she has failed? To me it's a shame, and unfortunately, we midwives play a part in it. For example, when midwives change shifts, I hear them say, "In that room we have Michal, she gave birth like a champ, we didn't hear a peep out of her, well done!" or, "Here is Shiran, she didn't take any pain medication, what an incredible woman." No one says, "Here is Yehudit, she had an epidural with half an inch of dilation, I'm so proud of her."

You'd think that the pain and dealing with it is all there is and all that matters. What do we know about the other challenges that this woman has faced that have nothing to do with pain at all? Maybe she was sexually abused as a child and, for her, the fact that she did not fall apart mentally or emotionally is equivalent to climbing Mount Everest. Maybe she went through some sort of domestic abuse and deals daily with a terrible reality that drains her completely and she simply does not have the energy to deal with physical pain during birth. Maybe her mother died a month ago. Maybe she suffers from anxiety because she has a child at home who is disabled as a result of a problem during his birth. There are a million and one things that this woman could be facing and we look only at "how she coped with the pain" and then evaluate her performance accordingly.

And since I have already brought up the subject, I have another thing to say about this. Sometimes women tell me, "I don't have good veins," when I am trying to find a vein to connect the IV to.

"Good veins for what?" I ask. For needles? After all, they are not designed for needles. They were made for returning blood from the body back to the heart, and they are doing that job very well!

Well, anyway, I gave her a good talking-to. I was a little less loaded than the things I wrote here, but that was because she was in labor and needed to keep her oxytocin levels high. Then I examined her. She was 3 centimeters dilated and I had a great feeling that this birth was going to happen here and now. The head was low and the pelvis was wide, and there was plenty of space for the baby to go through. I told her this and she asked for an epidural. At this point, her contractions were really strong and at short intervals and I believed that by the time the anesthesiologist arrived she would probably progress even more.

After she had her epidural, I checked her again at her request, and she was now 6 centimeters dilated. We were very happy, so we talked a bit about breastfeeding; we tried to think about what would help her this time, compared to her previous birth. There was a good atmosphere in the room, and this was boosted even further when her mother arrived. A doctor who examined her said that in his view, she had a great pelvis and there was no impediment for giving birth vaginally. He also said that the website calculator was not an appropriate statistical reference.

She progressed very quickly but then the fetal monitor started to show heart rate decelerations, which were quite severe and long-lasting - so much so that a doctor rushed into our room every couple of minutes. The woman felt discouraged again and said that maybe it was better to go into surgery and be done with it.

"Why should I go through all that and then go to surgery anyway?" she said.

But her family and I kept on encouraging her.

And then, she was at full dilation and started to push. At one point, a doctor came into the room and said, "Good! Now surely we won't go to surgery. Worst case, we'll have to vacuum." Two minutes later, a different doctor came in and said, "Just so you know, worst case, we will have to go to surgery since there is no possibility of using the vacuum."

It would have been funny if it wasn't so sad.

Now, the second phase of a vaginal birth with an epidural may take up to three hours; actually, it may take even more, but that's the time frame allowed by the hospital before an intervention. I knew that we had time, so I assured her that we didn't need to rush and that she shouldn't worry if things progressed slowly. Suddenly, a doctor informed me that in fact she had only two hours and not three, because she is a post-dissection patient with a large baby and variable deceleration in the fetal pulse, and he is not going to give her three hours. Damn it! That meant she had only another half hour.

I went back to her, turned off the epidural, even though she begged me not to, and we went to work. And work it did, quite fast to be honest, and in exactly two hours from achieving full dilation and perhaps only forty-five minutes since we started pushing, our charming 'big baby,' who weighted exactly nine pounds, was born. Within fifteen minutes, he was sucking enthusiastically on his mother's breast, and was still doing so when I saw her two weeks later.

Throughout the rest of that day, I walked as if I was on high heels, with my neck stretched high like a swan and a big ol' grin on my face. I felt as if it had been me who had given birth and I was so happy. I understand now how women feel when they have a successful vaginal delivery after a C-section. I think it was a corrective experience for both of us, and I'm really glad I got to attend this birth.

By the way, they named the child Dan, after Dana. That was a first for me...

The woman in Room 6 is a victim of domestic violence. She denies it, of course, and her family denies it, but the frightened look in her eyes betrays the truth. Her mother is with her, quiet as a shadow, her face clouded with thoughts, her steps hesitant; she makes me wonder about her own life with her husband's family. The husband threatens his wife and the medical staff, saying we should not dare to even think of giving her an epidural, but he eventually leaves. Later he will return, engulfed by a strong smell of booze, but in the meantime, the atmosphere in the delivery room lightens in his absence.

The woman is not quite in labor yet. She is having almost no contractions, perhaps one every twenty minutes or so, and no dilation at all, but she cries and screams all the time; tearing up and whimpering in between contractions, and screaming like a wounded animal during contractions. After a few hours of this, the staff has become uneasy around her. They suggest that she take a hot shower, have a massage, take analgesics... but she refuses everything. The team begins to resent this. Why doesn't she want anything for the pain? Does she enjoy suffering like this?

And I think to myself, finally this woman has a real, legitimate reason to scream and shout, cry and wail. What a rare opportunity for her to unload everything that weighs on her and burdens her soul. And I do not know whether to be happy for her or sad, and finally I decide to just be there for her.

❖ ❖ ❖

This next woman is barely more than a child herself. She is only nineteen years old, and doesn't really know who's who and what's what in this thing called labor. At any given moment, she clings to her husband, her mother or me. She doesn't allow us to let go of her hand, and she won't let anyone leave the room. It hurts her, it is hard for her, it takes too long, and it frightens her too much. After many hours, she gives birth. This is her first birth and it is long and debilitating; like parting the Red Sea.

Finally she lies back, on a clean bed, with a little bundle of joy in her hands, wondering what she should do next. I suggest she try to nurse the baby and she asks for help.

"I have no idea what to do now," she admits. I love helping women to breastfeed and so I'm about to take on the task willingly. But suddenly something stops me and I tell her, a little harshly, "Sorry, I have to finish a few things. I can't help you right now." And I go away.

I really am a little busy but not that much, and after a couple of minutes her husband appears, also young and nervous, asking me to help her. He says that she "really, really does not know what to do." I promise I'll get to her in a little while, but I'm not rushing. Something in me wants to run and stick the nipple in that baby's mouth, but something also tells me to wait one more minute.

Finally, after ten minutes or so, I get to her room, and see a happy mother. Her eyes beam with joy as she looks lovingly at her nursing baby, and she is filled with pride. Her eyes meet mine and she declares, "I did it!"

❖ ❖ ❖

This woman is already experienced in giving birth. It's her fifth birth and she always had good, empowering births. She is not accompanied by her husband, because he is at home, keeping an eye on the little ones, but the delivery room is quiet and I can sit next to her almost the entire time. She is very withdrawn, composed and concentrated in some internal process she is going through. Occasionally she makes those beautiful sounds, high-pitched at first but they get lower as the birth progresses.

It's late at night. I'm tired and I allow myself to close my eyes. My ears still listen to the fetal heart rate monitor and my head still processes everything and makes sure that everything is fine, but other parts of me are starting to sail along with this woman into the ether, where she is now to be found.

I start making sounds just like her. Bit by bit, I loosen up and sometimes make other noises that miraculously create great harmonies with the sounds she makes. I touch her and massage her back, and occasionally feel where it is appropriate to touch now, how hard to press and when to just gently lay my hand. Every time I touch her she hums and confirms, "Yes, that's exactly the spot."

I suddenly know that birth is near. It's not a guess, I really know. I whisper to her that her birth is coming up and slowly begin to organize everything; without noise and without interrupting her.

Into this stillness, a baby is born. The woman is crying and I feel tears in my eyes as well. Usually this does not happen to me, probably because I focus on other things, such as the fetal monitor, and because I'm busy with other births as well, or maybe because I'm not really part of the process but only watching it from the side. This time though, I really am a part of it, and I'm excited and happy and feeling that this woman, whom I only met a few hours ago, is like a family member or a good friend. I feel that we are soul mates. That's strange, because now as I write I don't even remember what she looks like or even her name, but I know that something was created between us and that this something continues to exist.

When something is missing

How can one fall in love with a woman giving birth, when some fundamental connection is lacking? When "lacking connection" is actually drastically underestimating the situation? Imagine a woman who is the complete opposite of you; totally different, and not in an interesting kind of way, but different in the sense of having a completely different mindset and worldview. Sometimes it's a woman who is very rude, demanding, annoying, needy, oblivious, or even outright hostile. Imagine a person you really do not like, maybe even despise. Now, imagine this person and imagine you need to help her give birth.

You need to help her and to be everything for her – you need to be supportive, maternal, loving, receiving, caring and encouraging. How do you do it? And let's add another layer, let's imagine that maybe she also has a husband or a family that is like her, and every time you enter the room you shudder.

I'm writing here of very extreme cases of course, but there are also cases of women who are not very annoying and not very daunting, but who are just not really my cup of tea. I need to take care of them and they need to be loved as well.

Yes, I have not only to take care of them professionally but to really love them. Actually, not love, but fall in love, completely; to want the best for them and to give them the best in me. At least that's what I think.

Obviously you cannot judge them; you cannot flinch or be disgusted; you cannot be angry with them for what they are or who they are. I can do these things perhaps in another place and another time, but not while I'm their midwife. They did not come here to get that from me.

I find that this is really not an easy task. Sure, it is easy to say, "I love all of humanity." Well, it's true, I love the 'idea' of humanity; I love the potential of human beings; their possibilities and capabilities, and that glimmer of promise within us; I love what we can be for each other, and for the world, and for God. I really love the idea. But the reality is not always close to what was promised. So I develop all kinds of techniques that help me to love them... to fall in love with them.

I tell myself that what I do not like in this particular person is not the essence of that individual, but things that got stuck to her during the course of her life, perhaps even as a baby or a small child. I tell myself that these are the effects of the culture in which we live, not the person herself. I try to imagine this person growing up in a loving environment, and how she would turn out. I try to understand her, to be in her place, to remind myself that I really do not know anything about her. I do not know what her desires, secret thoughts, cries and dreams are.

So many times I have been surprised at what dwells inside people after peeling away a bit of their outer shell and exposing what is hidden under all those layers of cynicism or rudeness or degeneration. I myself was covered in similar layers until a few years ago, and shedding them is a fascinating process for me too; to reveal that gentleness that is so vulnerable in this world. It is much easier to hide inside a shell and be protected. It is less painful that way.

I almost always make a deliberate effort to touch the woman, trying to feel the person inside by caressing a hand, a shoulder, her hair. Somehow, touch bypasses barriers that the brain and eyes put up before us. I search for the beauty in her face. It is very important for me to see beauty in every person, and it's especially easy to succeed in childbirth, when women are so beautiful.

And I try not to run away from it. When I turn up for a shift where it's clear to everyone that the woman in Room 3 is a "handful," I immediately volunteer to take care of her, if I'm not completely exhausted. I then try to be with her as much as possible - especially if it's hard for me - until I fall in love. And by the time I fall in love, she is ready to give birth and everything just falls into place. And because sometimes the woman may give birth really quickly, I have to fall in love really quickly. This is apparently a kind of ability that one can develop.

I still have difficulties sometimes with this rapid forced intimacy, a bit like an arranged marriage, where the couple did not really see each other before the ceremony, and then they find themselves alone in a room having to love each other and have romantic intimacy. And here I am, just like this couple, having to know this woman, and whoops, to touch her most intimate parts; even more than that, I am about to become part of the most exciting and important moment in her life, and not as a bystander, but as someone with a significant role to play. Not that I think that my role has to be significant, but a lot of times that's how it turns out, for better or worse.

And being really shy by nature, I don't easily know how to bond with people. I am terrible at small talk, and prefer to stay quiet if I don't feel really confident. Not to mention my general embarrassment about discussing sexuality; up until I was twenty-six, I had never said the word "period" out loud. When talking about genitalia in nursing school I blushed like a ripe tomato and just the thought of touching other people's bodies, let's say the chest, made me withdraw into myself and curl up like some kind of pastry.

But nursing school effectively cured most of these issues - this is another reason why I think everyone should really learn to be a nurse - and after I had washed some people confined to bed, inserted some catheters and administered more than a few enemas, this shyness, at least the one connected to touching other people's bodies, disappeared. And the rest I continue to deal with all the time and am making real improvements; at least I think so.

This may give the impression that a midwife has to be warm and loud and funny and outgoing and extroverted. Actually, no, this ability is just a tool. A midwife should also know how to keep quiet, to blend in with the background and to be an extra in a play, and not just the star. She has to be amusing with a woman who likes humor and quiet with one who doesn't. I always tiptoe into the delivery room (metaphorically), and try to understand with whom I am dealing today. What is suitable and what is not; at what speed should I talk and move; how loud should I speak and whether to make any sound at all; should I encourage or remain silent; should I hug or give some space; what tone of voice should I use to inspire confidence in this woman; should I be with her in the room as much or as little as possible; should I try to encourage the husband to take part or let him find his own rhythm or perhaps even encourage him to wait outside the room because that's what the woman secretly wants...

So many questions, and I have to get all my answers in just a few minutes or even seconds. And sometimes, when I have several women to take care of, I feel like a juggler, throwing balls and having to catch them all the time without getting confused...having to change the way I act within seconds.

It's such a good exercise. I do not know what for, but it's a good exercise.

A strange world

The elevator from the maternity ward opens and out comes an old lady. She has a limp in her foot, a hump on her back and thick glasses that barely conceal the cloudiness of the cataracts in her eyes.

"I bet she came to get monitored," I joke quietly when suddenly this old lady comes up and hands me a hospital admission sheet.

"I came to get monitored," she announces in a pleasant voice, and I almost swallow my tongue and choke. Tactfully, I lead her to a room and hook her up to a monitor. It turns out that she is pregnant with a baby girl, and that this is her first pregnancy. Ten years of fertility treatments finally bore fruit and at the distinguished age of sixty-three, Sarah became pregnant. It is hard for her to get on the bed and hard for her to get off. In the past two years, she fell twice and broke the femur in both legs. In general, everything is difficult, but not so bad, because it is a miracle that she is pregnant. She has been waiting for this for a long time, her family is happy and her husband is happy, and she will receive a lot of support and everything will be just fine.

What a strange world. Many children are looking for parents, and many parents are looking for children, but those parents do not want other people's children, they want their own. Even if the price is endless fertility treatments (a few months ago, a baby was born in our ward after seventeen years of intensive fertility treatments), even if it's at the age of sixty-three, even if the pregnancy endangers the woman, or goes against all logic. And the truth is, a lot of times it's not really their children, but the fertilized eggs of others. Hardly any woman over the age of forty-five gets pregnant with her own eggs. Pregnancy at this age is almost always the outcome of an egg donation, and sometimes also a surrogate mother. So if the child is not the woman's biological child, what is it all about anyway? Sometimes the problem is the husband. Men want to have their own child, not another man's child, because if it's another man's child then their biological instinct is not to raise it, but rather to eat it. Ah, sorry, we are not lions but people. But still, if you have a child, then it is better that it is yours, all yours.

I know that these are rough generalizations. I would like to apologize to all those men who lovingly raise adopted children; I know there are a lot of those. I also would like to apologize to all those mothers who eagerly wait for a child. I'm not underestimating your longing or your love. I too wanted to have a child that I bore and did not want to give up on the idea of pregnancy and birth. I just think of this unbalanced equation of children who are yearning for parents and parents that yearn for a child, but only for one that is biologically theirs.

Sometimes the way we work seems so surreal and absurd

The night began with a busy but pleasant shift. We were two midwives on duty and Marcella, a nursing assistant, who is basically as good as a midwife, if not better. We were hoping for the best - that is, that there would not be too much work - because, after all, we were only two midwives.

At the beginning of the shift, I ran into a woman whom I had cared for throughout my entire shift the previous day. She had been induced, due to the fact that her waters had broken five days earlier. It turned out that during her previous birth, I had also taken care of her and had helped her with breastfeeding. I didn't remember, but she did, and so a certain relationship began to develop between us.

During the previous shift, she didn't progress at all, but when we arrived for the night shift she had gone into labor and one of the evening shift midwives had assured her that she would give birth within an hour. Well, it took only half an hour in the end, and it was great.

Unfortunately, this uplifting and otherwise uncomplicated birth was followed by the placenta not being delivered intact. The woman was bleeding and we had to perform a manual extraction of the missing piece under general anesthesia. About a month earlier, we had moved into a new delivery room and I still hadn't used the new operating theater, so I found myself running around like a headless chicken trying to find a long list of items required for an intra-uterine examination: drugs, needles, syringes, sleeves, gloves, antiseptic, antibiotics, birth kit, stitching kit, IV pole, stickers for the monitor, a bag of fluids, and so on and so on.

After this little drama ended, we had a steady trickle of women who came to the delivery room. For some reason, they were all in week twenty-seven and all experiencing premature contractions (Did I mention the rule of threes already?) After that, it was calm again.

At 4 AM, the heavens opened up and women began to pour into the delivery room. One woman came in from the maternity ward with 8 centimeters dilation. We thought to ourselves, no problem, we can still handle the rush. I was supposed to take care of her while the other midwife handled the three women who were having premature contractions and one woman with an epidural. Then another woman came to the ER with 8 centimeters dilation. No problem, the other midwife said she could handle it as well. Then another woman came from the maternity ward with 6 centimeters dilation. Well, we hoped they wouldn't all give birth at the same time, but still basically thought we could manage it all somehow. Then another woman came from the ER with 3 centimeters dilation and a delivery that was progressing rapidly.

So now what? Should we try to manage or should we call for help? We decided that we'd try to manage. The time was 5 AM anyway, so there wasn't really anyone we could call. We didn't felt like waking anyone up, and in truth we also didn't have the time to sit by the phone.

Meanwhile, the woman who had come from the maternity ward had given birth, but her placenta had not been born and she was bleeding from her cervix -- but we were still in control. Then another woman turned up with 8 centimeters dilation. Help!!! At this stage, we called Nili, our devoted head midwife, for help. She lives the closest and is always ready to come and save us. There was a moment when five women were shouting at exactly the same time from every room in the ward: Ohhhh! Eeeee! Ahh! Ahawo!!!

Ahihihi!! They were all progressing so quickly, without epidurals and without analgesics, and the three of us were bumping into each other while running from point A to point B or from point B to point C. It was just weird and we all split our sides with laughter and kept on running.

And during all this, I thought to myself, what kind of a job is this? Am I a midwife at all? Maybe I'm just someone who sticks stickers, fills out forms, takes blood tests, checks dilations, takes notes, opens birth kits, delivers babies, registers births and moves on to the next delivery. This is not midwifery – this is project management! And during all this time, I think to myself, *make it that nothing will happen…that we won't miss anything… that everyone involved will survive this night unscathed and that no more women will come in, because if they do we will really fall apart*... And then in came another woman, and we did not fall apart, because we are strong and resilient, and have you ever heard of a nurse, let alone a midwife, falling apart or caving in? We have to manage, never leave unfinished work for the next shift, never complain or whine and, of course, never forget anything; more accurately, never forget to write anything down, because, "if it's not written down, you haven't done it!"

It was interesting to try and identify which woman should be approached first from their tone of voice and their shouting. A woman sounds completely different when she is just having contractions compared to when the baby is about to be born. It's a pretty accurate science and much more reliable than the monitor, for example. So it happened that all of us - the three midwives, Marcella, the nursing the assistant, and the doctor - came to the same room, all at once, after we heard that unmistakable sound, only to see the baby's head emerging. The most agile of us put on gloves and received the delivery and the rest turned to care for the other women. I guess that's how a perineum feels at birth; it expands and expands and constantly thinks it can't get any wider, but then it finds that it can...

In the end, everything went well and all of the mothers were, miraculously, satisfied and didn't stop praising us. I don't know why. What's so praiseworthy about a midwife who says, "Hello, I'm Dana, call me when the baby comes out, bye"...?

After I had dragged myself back home and crawled into bed with Eitan and Ya'ara, I found that I couldn't sleep because of all the adrenaline in my body. Then Ya'ara woke up and after I breastfed her, she asked, "How many births were there tonight?" and when I answered, "Seven," she opened her eyes wide in amazement and said, "Wow! That's a lot of babies!"

"Yes, that's a lot" I told her, and she was delighted and happy. And then I fell asleep.

May you know no grief

Luma is one of the midwives in our staff. She is a Bedouin, who was born in a small and distant village. On Monday night, her brother, Mahmoud, was killed in a car accident. His two small children were with him in the car, but they were unharmed, physically at least.

So I went to the funeral in Luma's village – well, not to the funeral exactly, as Muslim women do not participate in funerals – but we went to visit the mourners' house. Her village is a beautiful place with lots of anemones and ancient oak trees, and everything is so green and quiet; too quiet. I got there and began searching for the mourners' house. I asked two elderly women I saw on the street if they were going there and if I could join them, and we walked silently together the rest of the way.

Upon our arrival, it seemed to me that all of the women of the village were there – inside, outside... Almost all of them wore a *hijab* and dark clothes, and were very serious. As we approached the house, I heard a whisper that went through the crowd of women like wildfire, "Luma, Luma." Somehow they realized I had come to see Luma...

They all encouraged me to go up a narrow stairway, which was filled with many, many women looking at me with piercing eyes, leaving only a very narrow path for me to go up or down. I went and found Luma, surrounded by other midwives, all hugging and very serious, and I felt again the sense of family that exists among our staff; we really support each other through thick and thin. I too hugged Luma, trying without words to convey what I felt and all the love and support I had for her.

I recalled the funeral of Myrna, a midwife who was killed in a car accident four years ago, when I was still an intern; and the funeral of Miriam, which happened exactly one year ago. She was a cleaning lady who had worked in our delivery room for twenty-five years and was killed in a car accident the day before she retired; So many funerals and so much pain.

Then I went to console Mahmoud's wife for the death of her husband, and she said to me, "May you know no grief, and may we meet only on happy occasions." She seemed to me like a remarkable woman, strong and composed, as if she had already decided not to let this break her.

Then, on the way home, I thought about what she said to me – *May you know no grief* - and I thought to myself that I actually do want to know grief in my lifetime. I want to know grief and joy and loss and frustration -- and the feeling of overcoming it all. I want to know the full spectrum of emotions felt by human beings; that's why I came here, to this world, to feel it all and to learn from everything. Many times, I feel so young and immature because I have barely experienced anything in this lifetime. Sometimes I feel like things are not real until it doesn't turn your stomach and sometimes I wonder if it is not a matter of character and attitude. I know people who have gone through the same things I have, but their experience of it all was quite different. I'm not used to looking at problems as difficulties and I don't consider anything I went through to have been traumatic. Even death does not scare me, except for my daughter's death, which I hope and pray will come long after I die.

"So how many people are allowed in the delivery room?"

We get asked this question a lot. In most hospitals, the number of family members or friends who are allowed to be with the woman during birth is limited to one or two. We, on the other hand, don't limit the number of people; perhaps because it does not quite fit the type of population we care for. How can you say that only one family member can go into the delivery room? Who will it be? The husband? What's his connection to this childbirth anyway? Maybe the mother? The mother-in-law? The older sister? And what about little sister? The sister-in-law? And the brother-in-law? And the woman's best friend? And the other best friend, who also came because she gave birth two months ago and has lots of good advice? What about the maternal grandfather? Or the woman's maternal uncle? And her little brother? He is also very interested in what is going on. And we haven't mentioned the aunt yet, or the mother's friend who happens to work at the hospital and who heard that her friend's daughter is about to give birth and was curious to see how she deals with labor. In short, why limit the number of people to just one or two, you wouldn't want to offend anyone, and if they came from far away then why not give them something to drink, or something to eat, or more than just something...

And everyone wants to hear the woman's screams, click with their tongues, *tsk tsk tsk*, and say, "Poor thing, she is in so much pain!" and "Just give her an epidural" or "What a wonderful midwife!" or "What a lovely doctor." And every time I leave the delivery room people I have never seen before ask me, "So how dilated is she?" Sure, let's all stand in between her legs. I try to preserve the privacy of the mother, but the husband doesn't hesitate, walks outside and calls out to everyone that she is 8 centimeters dilated. "Mom, Limor, call everyone in. She is 8 centimeters dilated!" he hollers down the hall.

As the baby comes out, the mother strategically places her cell phone right between her daughter's legs, to broadcast the birth live to all those relatives who, for some reason, were unable to come. And everyone wants to see the baby, hear him cry, comment that he looks exactly like his mother or father or older brother or no one at all. And if we need to perform CPR on the baby, wow, let them all come and see.

What's the deal with these annoying delivery room staff, who ask us politely to wait in the waiting room so the doctor can treat the newborn baby? And now the staff claim they are "upset" - such nerve they have. After all, we are her family! We just want to see the woman. So what if the staff are still stitching her up, we just want to say hello because we've been here for a long time and are dying to go home already.[47]

---

47 A few words about privacy at birth: Birth is as intimate process as the baby's conception. Almost the same hormones that get secreted into our body during intercourse are the ones that trigger the birth, produce the woman's contractions, help to overcome pain, and encourage the bonding between the mother and her newborn. Imagine that you are two people trying to reach orgasm, when suddenly your parents, siblings, friends and distant relatives are present in the room. There is not much chance it will happen that way. The natural process of birth requires privacy, it requires a sense of security, it requires calmness from that part of our minds that likes to ask questions all the time, is interested in what's going on and wants to run things. Think of your cat. When she is about to give birth she enters the darkest, most comfortable closet and does it there, in private. We are not cats, but when our sense of privacy and security at birth is undermined, the secretion of hormones in our body and the natural process of birth is delayed or stopped. So you should give the mother some privacy, you should let her drift into her own world, not ask too many questions, not offer too many suggestions, not visit if you do not have to, not turn on the lights. You should let the body do what it knows best, and believe me, it knows best. Our mind, the thing that makes us smart, that helped us establish our glorious career, the one that keeps all of our thoughts and opinions and notions, can go to sleep for a few hours.

Having your mother in the delivery room

A woman giving birth for the first time is lying in bed, all bleary-eyed after not sleeping for thirty-two hours, her hair disheveled and her skin sweaty. She is exhausted and in pain, hungry but nauseous, barely remembers who or where she is, and with each contraction she seems more tired and even more exhausted.

And here comes her mother. She slept all night in her bed, woke up and put on her best clothes to greet her new grandson, put on makeup and combed her hair, donned jewelry and sprayed herself with perfume. She is freshness personified. She looks at her daughter with a loving and compassionate look and says:

"**I** gave birth to you in five minutes."

And then thrusting the knife deeper:

"And in my day, there was no such thing as an epidural."

A perfect child, that's what they all want

Everyone wants a perfect child; a cute little thing with big eyes, preferably blue, and definitely two of them; a head full of locks, a sweet smile and some dimples. Other people can raise all those less-than-perfect children, say, children with one kidney or a hole in their heart; children with cleft lips, dwarfism, six fingers... But not here. Our children need to be perfect.

So we check all the time. There are those who start even before marriage, checking if there is a genetic match between the families so there won't be a chance that, Heaven forbid, they will bear children with some genetic disease. Others are less strict about this and wait until they are pregnant. Then they begin a chain of endless blood tests, scans, then some more scans, and maybe a repeat scan because the previous scan showed a small echogenic spot in the heart, and then a nuchal translucency and amniocentesis.

It turns out that Israel leads the world in the number of tests performed during pregnancy, and the abortion rate is the highest, due to the findings from these tests. Well, if it is a life-threatening defect, or one that causes severe mental retardation or some other serious problems, I can understand it, and even identify with the parents. However when they terminate a pregnancy at week twenty-one because of a cleft lip, an aesthetic defect that does not hinder a person from having a full and happy life...

Everyone wants a perfect child and would do almost anything to get one; as if there was some kind of insurance we can buy to guarantee such a thing. After all, anything can happen. Someone marries a perfect husband and two years later he has an accident and becomes paralyzed, or perhaps he becomes schizophrenic. Someone else has a wonderful baby girl, genetically she is a model of perfection, but during birth not enough oxygen reached the brain, and now the child is suddenly not so perfect. Too bad they don't come with a receipt.

The Choice

It's Friday night and I am caring for a young woman giving birth for the first time. We have connected and feel comfortable with each other. One of the times I go into the delivery room, I find a familiar face: an older woman, whom I helped give birth two months ago at an early stage of pregnancy, with a pair of still-born twin girls.

"What are you doing here?" I ask her, surprised.

"This is our daughter giving birth," she says with a smile.

That is, this was not exactly her daughter, because she has no children. This was actually the daughter of her husband. She had married late in her life, to a widower, a father of five, and they had been trying to have a child since, with no success.

I remember the special bond that we shared during her birth, the shared pain and the intimacy that had been created despite, or perhaps because, of the difficult circumstances. Then I look at her and there is a kind of illusion - for if I look for just a second and then turn my head away, I notice nothing special. She just looks at me and smiles. But if I look at her a little longer, I see something change. Her face turns red, and her eyes glisten.

And I find I have a choice here: I could look away and leave the room, carry on with my own business, ignore what I just saw in that brief moment and doubt that there was anything there at all. Maybe I was just imagining it? And besides, who has time for all this...? Or, I could stay. And by stay I mean keep looking at her, letting our eyes meet, letting our souls meet, letting our hearts get closer. And then, the moment her eyes brim over with tears, to hug her and not let go until she decides to let go, until she feels it's enough, even if it is a very long hug.

For me, this moment, this choice between leaving the room and being there for her, or not necessarily for her but for life, is a choice between living, truly living, and merely surviving.

After two years in the delivery room, most of the time I still feel as if I'm just at the beginning.

Most of our delivery room midwives have worked in this business more years than I've lived, and upon encountering such vast experience, it is hard not to feel as if I'm just a novice. And yet, sometimes, I feel like I've earned my stripes; that I too have the ability to sense what's going on rather than just think that I do. Sometimes it is like that and sometimes it is the other way around. And as strange as it may sound, sometimes midwives with thirty years of experience consult with me. That's part of what I like in midwifery -- the humility that it makes us feel when facing the world. Because we do not really know what will happen or when, and can only try to guess and then still be surprised in most cases.

Today I took care of a woman giving birth for the first time. She had been in the process of induction for several days but with no results. When I met her she had one centimeter dilation. Then her contractions became more crowded and she slipped into it and it was no longer possible to talk to her. She yelled and cried and didn't respond to any of our questions. At first, I gave her massages and it helped, but after some time she did not want to be touched anymore. She was so beautiful, not in the "regular" sense of the word but beautiful from the inside; a woman you can see is clean, without all the nonsense, like a child. By the way, I do think that every woman is beautiful during childbirth, even more than on her wedding day,[48] since at her wedding she is beautiful but perhaps doesn't quite look like her usual self, and at birth she is even more herself than usual.

And so she drifted away, from the short and shallow contractions into the deep waters, and then into this ocean of pain that sometimes feels as if it is about to drown you in it along with anyone that is with you. I had some difficult moments with this. Over the previous two days I had worked two insane shifts and I felt that on top of my physical fatigue I had no capacity for other people's pain. But I talked with myself about it and resisted the urge to run away. I jumped into the water with her, and despite it being cold at first, I got used to it; it even made us feel good in a strange way. After an hour, I examined her and she was fully dilated.

The second stage of birth wasn't easy either. After each contraction, she cried a lot, begged me to make it stop and said that she can't take it anymore. Within a few contractions, her husband and I had already developed an encouraging drill and as time passed, it became easier and she just fell asleep in between contractions. She had long breaks between contractions, which was great. By the way, many times during the second stage of birth there are suddenly long breaks between contractions, which are a wonderful change after the intensity of the previous stage. The woman can rest and recover her strength after trying to push; she can sometimes even fall asleep and gather her strength that way. There is simply no limit to the genius of this process.

So let's get back to that beautiful woman. She pushed and pushed, and we encouraged and supported her, and the baby did his bit and moved slowly towards us, progressing and retracting, progressing and retracting, like it is with all first births. He showed us

48 There is a saying in Hebrew that a woman is always beautiful on her wedding day.

his long black hair and retreated again until the moment he revealed himself in all his sweet glory. I think that during the first hour after birth, the woman was still a little bit in shock from the intensity that just grabs you like a tornado. She scarcely said a word and instead just concentrated on breathing and recovering her strength. After a while, she began to smile and breastfeed, and said she had had the dreamiest birth.

Being who you are

A well-dressed woman walked calmly into our reception. I was deeply impressed by her perfect hairdo and delicate makeup. She was perfumed, wearing small pearl earrings, her clothes were perfectly pressed and she had on a beautiful pair of high heels. It was four in the morning so that it was a bit strange. She was having contractions and this was her fourth birth. I tried to guess where she could have come from to be dressed so nicely; maybe some festive event that ended late at night? Maybe her plane had just landed? I could not think of any plausible option, but after a few minutes, the mystery was solved. She said she had been asleep, and suddenly her waters broke, so she got dressed and came straight to the delivery room. "Well," I said to myself, "there are people who dress nicely every time they leave the house."

After I examined her, it turned out that she was in active labor and had 5 centimeters dilation. She did not seem to be in much pain, despite her dilation and the crowded contractions on the monitor. When I told her that, she nodded and said she wasn't particularly in pain right now but that in previous births it began to hurt later on, so she wanted an epidural. I asked her if she wanted to maybe try and have a natural birth, but she laughed and said that soon she would begin to act like a bitch and bark at everyone, and then she would begin to behave like a cat and wail and cry and she thought she would rather act like a person and give birth that way.

She sounded very convincing so I immediately called the anesthesiologist to give her an epidural, and all the while the woman was perfectly calm, well-groomed and elegant, just as she was from the moment she walked in. After the anesthesiologist went away we talked a bit and she told me that she was an HMO family physician, and I could actually imagine her giving prescriptions and checking patients, with the exact same clothes and the same beautiful hairdo.

The birth progressed very quickly, after all it was her fourth delivery, and in less than half an hour after receiving the epidural, she gave birth. She almost did not push at all, or at least you couldn't see her pushing, since everything was done so elegantly, and when the baby was born I made sure to wipe him clean before I laid him on her. There was great excitement in the room; she and her husband were very happy and when they pulled out the camera and I offered to take their photograph, the woman asked her husband for her purse, took out a small mirror and comb, arranged her hair, put on lipstick and only then gave me the green light to take the picture. It was a little funny, and a little weird, but somehow it was also in perfect harmony. The woman gave birth the same way she lives her life, and that was the best way for her and therefore also the best way for me too.[49]

---

49 Gayle Peterson, in her book 'Birthing Normally', writes: "As a woman lives, so shall she give birth."

Somewhere out there, there's a hug for me

This week I met a lovely woman in the delivery room during her third birth. She reminded me that, during her first birth, I had been her midwife, and she refreshed my memory regarding those minute things that may sound bland and boring to an outsider, but which are the crucial details that make up the story of any woman's process of giving birth: when her waters broke, and what did she do; when she arrived at the hospital, and how much pain she was in... and the truth is that I can listen to these stories almost indefinitely.

Then she told me, "You know, never in my life will I forget the hug you gave me while I was in severe pain. That hug has stayed with me ever since, and I sometimes still remember it."

"Wow," I think to myself. "Somewhere out there in the world, there's a hug I gave, that's floating around and I am not even aware of it."

This is how we live in this world; spreading words, looks, deeds... and hugs. Once we do these things, they are no longer ours -- they take on lives of their own. Some of these acts become significant for another person, and will continue to live on, in and through them. Will my hug come back to me someday? Maybe on my last day, after I die?

This short sentence uttered by this woman changed the way I perceive the world. Now, she walks around with my hug and I walk around with her words.

Late night contemplations

I'm with a woman in the delivery room, late at night. Everyone is sleeping and the streets are dark and quiet. I touch her; hold her hand, whisper to her. I watch her as she sheds her skin and lets her guard down, as she lets loose her inhibitions, as her boundaries are breached and she reaches the highest peaks of her life. I am with her and think that, basically, at the beginning of each person's path, there is a birth; this is how life begins. Every birth is a point in time, but this point involves a whole life story; a story about love, a story about fear, a story about overcoming, about pain and about hope -- a life story.

So many people come to this earth, so many new lives, and each one is unique and special - there will never be another like it. And I stand here, at this gate, through which life enters this place, and I get to see the private moments that almost always remain hidden and unnoticed by the rest of the world. And if I do not forget to look, I get to see the uniqueness of every woman, of every man, of every baby, of each and every birth.

I know that even though birth is a special once-in-a-lifetime experience for the woman, an experience she'll always remember, I probably won't remember it in a few days. I won't remember the woman's face; I won't remember her husband's name; I won't remember the baby's voice or his expression when he was born. I know I won't remember, and part of me mourns this. Part of me already knows, from the moment we first meet, that this is temporary, and says its farewell right there, at the start.

But there are parts of me that will never forget; those parts that bore witness to these unique and significant moments. Those parts of me that know that I was a part of this historic event, that, even though it probably will not be written about in tomorrow's newspaper, the world still changed a bit in its wake. And those moments shape and leave their mark on me, and I change a bit with each birth; getting a little bit wiser, more mature. I see things a little differently, like a tree that slowly puts down its roots and grows leaves. After a few years, one suddenly notices a big change has occurred.

Women give birth as they live, and birth is an opportunity to meet them as they are, to see life as it really is -- naked. And this meeting brings out the real me, who I really am, revealing my weaknesses and bringing to the surface all the insights I have gained, my inner resilience and the things I must improve in myself.

And sometimes these encounters drain me of all my juices, but this is the juice of life and I am happy that I have the opportunity to taste it. It is much tastier than Coca-Cola and much stronger than wine; it quenches the thirst better than water; and after you taste it, you can't settle for anything else.

www.ingramcontent.com/pod-product-compliance
Lightning Source LLC
Chambersburg PA
CBHW061435180526
45170CB00004B/1416
* 9 7 8 1 5 2 2 9 9 9 1 4 0 *